"Many patients suffering from multiple sclerosis have derived guidance and solice from Jeffrey Gingold's personal account, *Facing the Cognitive Challenges of Multiple Sclerosis.* His second publication, *Mental Sharpening Stones: Manage the Cognitive Challenges of Multiple Sclerosis*, builds on the success of the prior volume by adding personal reflections of other patients and advice on management by experts. These highly readable and practical books will be of immense benefit to patients, their families, and health professionals."

John Fleming, MD
Professor
Department of Neurology
University of Wisconsin
National Clinical Advisory Board for the NMSS

"One of the uplifting characteristics of our society is the fact that when professionals or elected officials fail to adequately address an issue of concern, the affected public will eventually rouse itself and fill the void. This is the case with cognitive dysfunction in multiple sclerosis, a common and sometimes major impairment whose recognition by the medical community has been deficient and its management sorely inadequate. Into this void steps Jeffrey Gingold with his latest book, *Mental Sharpening Stones.*

This thoughtful, articulate and timely volume will not only provide solace and counsel to many an MS patient, but is a must-read for any professional engaged in the management of this enigmatic condition, in which concealed disability often outweighs the revealed."

Dr. Joseph Herbert
Director of the MS Care Center
NYU Hospital for Joint Diseases

"This book is written by people who understand MS and what it's like to have mental disruptions due to this disease but you will go away with ideas and possibilities where before you might have only seen despair.

It's good to know we are not alone.

Now go write this down before you forget to remember to order this book. It's well worth every penny spent."

Liz Thompson
MSWorld
www.msworld.org

Mental Sharpening Stones

Mental Sharpening Stones

Manage the Cognitive Challenges of Multiple Sclerosis

Jeffrey N. Gingold

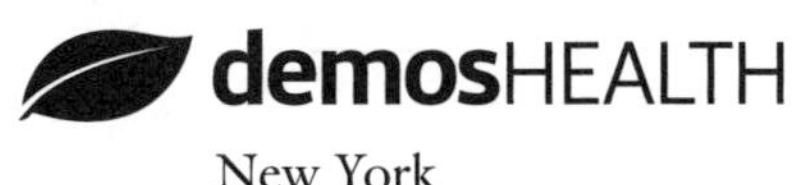

New York

Visit our web site at www.demosmedpub.com

Library of Congress Cataloging-in-Publication Data
Mental sharpening stones : manage the cognitive challenges of multiple sclerosis / [edited by] Jeffrey N. Gingold.
p. ; cm.
Includes bibliographical references and index.
ISBN-13: 978-1-932603-65-1 (pbk. : alk. paper)
ISBN-10: 1-932603-65-4 (pbk. : alk. paper)
1. Multiple sclerosis—Popular works. 2. Cognition disorders—Popular works. 3. Multiple sclerosis—Complications. I. Gingold, Jeffrey N.
[DNLM: 1. Multiple Sclerosis—complications. 2. Multiple Sclerosis—rehabilitation. 3. Adaptation, Psychological. 4. Cognition Disorders—prevention & control. 5. Cognition Disorders—rehabilitation. WL 360 M5495 2009]
RC377.M46 2009
616.8'34—dc22

2008017417

Made in the United States of America
08 09 10 11 5 4 3 2 1

Especially for Terri with her unwavering love and the ability to help me bridge the mental gaps to remain focused on true priorities—next to each other and holding hands—for Lauren and Meredith with their unselfish smiles and spontaneous hugs. For Mickey, too!

Contents

Preface

When I was seven years old, I realized that there was a ritual marking the end of a frigid Wisconsin winter and the anticipation of a warm summer. When my father switched the storm windows for screens, it openly brought the breeze and sounds of the neighborhood back into our home like a returning friend. Every few weeks, the morning calm was shattered by the sound of a clanging bell bouncing down the alley. The sound could be heard through my bedroom screen and rolled through our house, startling my Mom into action. It was the traveling knife sharpener.

One would have thought that the man would have quickly fled upon witnessing eight to ten women running down the alley toward him, all wielding handfuls of knives, scissors, and meat cleavers. Without any fear, he bravely stood his ground behind his pushcart. The wooden-handled cart was built around a large, stone-sharpening wheel, centered next to shelves stacked with smaller wheels and uniquely cut stones. As he rapidly spun the large stone on an axle, the man angled each knife against it, producing a scraping sound from stone grinding the metal to its sharpest edge. The line of women handed him their knives for cutting bread and steak, filleting fish, and hacking away at a 24-pound turkey.

Different knives required different stones, angles, and pressure against the turning wheel or hand-held stones. No one stone worked for all of the edges, and most often, each edge required more than one stone to bring out a fine edge. When our food was being ripped and not cut, my mother realized that a knife was losing its edge. It was simple—*using a sharp implement required less effort and was more effective.*

Unfortunately, not every person with multiple sclerosis (MS) is aware of the dulling impact of MS upon cognitive functions. These individuals may not fully understand that the once-sharp edges of their thoughts have been silently blunted—delayed or blocked by MS lesions. At the time of my diagnosis, I also didn't understand that this chronic disease would slow my thoughts and obscure recall. Even when I began to recognize that MS was interfering with my thoughts, I was unaware of any steps that I could take to preserve my cognitive connections.

Individuals dealing with MS may be confused and exasperated about where they left their car in the parking lot or unable to find the right words to complete their thoughts. Due to the effect of cognitive symptoms, the majority of people with MS may struggle to maintain their *presence of mind.* Their focus and ability to process information may be stalled or lost, tripped by a disconnection from thoughts. Concepts may be jammed by single- and multiple-task circumstances, suddenly and invisibly shut down—trapped in MS mental quicksand. How would you deal with it? What measures would you take to slow the encroachment of these confounding lapses in your thinking and to keep your mind sharp?

Each chapter in this book provides real-life techniques, inspired by people with MS and medical providers who have successfully adapted cognitive disconnection into cognitive flexibility and strength. By calling out the blunt cognitive obstacles that are being faced by themselves or the MS community, the writers have honestly and courageously shared their practical methods for pushing back against these disruptive and potentially disabling symptoms. By offering their successful coping methods, the writers believe that the strategies will assist people with MS to remain mentally active through sharpening their mental discipline. By pursuing cognitive techniques that invigorate the mind and facilitate better use of existing mental skills, people with MS will be enabled to draw a personal line against cognitive impediments.

The National Multiple Sclerosis Society recently stated that, "*Although it is among the more common symptoms of MS, cognitive dysfunction has suffered from neglect until relatively recently.*" The percentage of people who will face cognitive challenges may only be as surprising as the time that it has taken for the MS community to recognize the cognitive dysfunction as commonplace. Recent studies have established that 65% to 70% of people with MS will face some degree of cognitive symptoms. In the mainstream discussion of MS, there is a hunger for real-life examples of how people with MS may forestall and deal with cognitive hurdles. When their rational presence is distorted by the unimaginable memory twist of MS, how can they maintain their employment, preserve connections with family and friends, and otherwise pursue vital lives?

The writers in this book reach out to people with MS and their caregivers in an effort to convey that they are not relegated to silently endure disruption of their thoughts and stalled thinking. For those people with MS who have not yet faced cognitive impediments, they need not merely wait for the impact. Instead, they can learn mental-exercise tactics directly from those individuals who function with MS, but are not mutely waiting for cognitive setbacks. They exercise their minds with successful mental sharpening tools to stay ahead of any potential cognitive challenges.

When the MS community shares its cognitive experiences and coping strategies, the imparted knowledge is a powerful catalyst, promoting people's conversations with their doctors, therapists, family members, and friends—fostering a supportive network. The writers detail their knowledge of coping with and organizing against the cognitive challenges of MS, imparting the resiliency of people to fight back against the cognitive obstructions of MS.

These are real stories, born from and best told from personal experience.

The lesson of the sharpening stones echoed to me years later, as a member of the West Allis Speedskating Club. During my training sessions on the oval ice at the Pettit National Ice Center, I watched the focused determination of Olympians Dan Jansen and Bonnie Blair as they easily lapped me on the ice. Sensing that something was slowing down my glide in the straightaways, I skated off the ice and sat down on one of the blue wooden benches. Untying my skates, I took out a burr stone from my gear bag and began sliding it along the edges of the blades. The small stone began removing bits of metal burr left over from the two larger sharpening stones I had used the night before. The rough edges had been resisting the ice and reducing the ease of movement, slowing the glide.

Speedskating has taught me far more than that ice is slippery, hard, and cold. My last coach, Bob Fenn, taught me to always keep my blades razor sharp. Another speedskater, Mark, collapsed on the bench near me and asked if he could use by burr stone. Sharpening stones may be shared, but the technique can be personal. Either on ice or in processing thoughts, a dull edge can be ineffective and frustrating. Speedskaters may differ on the use of their stones, but they would agree that the personal technique to maintain sharpness is vital to holding your balance and focus and maximizing the use of your energy. After being diagnosed with MS, I found that principle rang true for living with MS, as well as for holding my edge on a sheet of ice.

Will a specific mix of physical and mental sharpening stones work for *all* people with MS? Probably not, and that is the point of this book. Just as no single disease-modifying medication is best for all people with MS, neither are the techniques for pushing back against the cognitive symptoms and disability of the disease. The tactics are as varied as the individuals. This book offers specific cognitive strategies that have proved successful for people with MS to maintain the sharpness in their thinking, as well as discusses the importance of proper understanding, diagnosis, and treatment of the mental-twister element of MS.

As a volunteer advocate and peer supporter for the National Multiple Sclerosis Society since 2001, I have had the opportunity to speak with numerous people with MS about their cognitive challenges. Although some people have discovered how to remain cognitively sharp by using their personal sharpening stones, most people have not. The writers in this book have joined forces to encourage the MS community to learn from each other and develop their own cognitive techniques, sharing their mental sharpening stones with others.

Jeffrey N. Gingold

Introduction

Iron rusts from disuse; stagnant water loses its purity and in cold weather becomes frozen; even so does inaction sap the vigor of the mind.

Leonardo da Vinci (1452–1519)
The Notebooks, 1, 2

Even for those individuals who are informed about the nature of multiple sclerosis (MS), they can hold stereotypes about the impact and appearance of the progressive disease. Whether or not you have been diagnosed with MS, it can be difficult for anyone to break through common notions about the disease and its impact on various people.

After watching his television talk show for many years, I found it strange meeting Phil Donahue, face-to-face. He was the keynote speaker at a luncheon fundraiser for the Wisconsin Chapter of the National Multiple Sclerosis Society. More than 700 people, including my wife, Terri, and I attended the event at the historic, 19th century Pfister Hotel in Milwaukee.

Mr. Donahue was admittedly uncomfortable when he began to speak. His comments followed a presentation regarding the castration of male mice in MS sex research. The image of the ill-fated mice was difficult to shake, but his presentation quickly took a more serious tone. A long-time member of Mr. Donahue's staff had recently died from complications related to MS. Mr. Donahue's shared thoughts, encouraging support of sex-based research, were genuine and heartfelt. He paused to suppress a choke in his voice as he reflected upon his friend's spirit and final days. Funding research to find an answer for MS was personal for Phil Donahue. We understood that he flew to Milwaukee to speak at the luncheon at his own cost.

After the function was complete, Terri and I were able to avoid the mass exodus from the seventh floor ballroom by heading for a remote elevator. As the doors opened, we found ourselves side by side with Mr. Donahue. It was a rare moment to directly thank someone for making such a difference.

"Mr. Donahue," I said, while we all continued to walk out of the elevator, "we just wanted to thank you for your comments and support of the Chapter's efforts. Because of your presence here, I understand that well over $200,000 was raised for MS research." He stopped walking, and we did too. As he turned toward us and smiled, he reached out and firmly shook my hand.

"Thank you very much for saying so," he said. It was time for a brief introduction.

"My name is Jeffrey Gingold and this is my wife, Terri," I said. He stepped forward and reached out to shake Terri's hand. While continuing to shake her hand, he slightly lowered the grasp, and, while maintaining eye contact with her, he softly spoke again.

"It's very nice to meet you," he said. "How are you doing?" His voice carried a soft bedside manner of understanding, in contrast to a casual hallway greeting.

"Doing fine," Terri answered. We talked about Milwaukee and that he would need to stop somewhere on the way back to the airport and bring some cheese back to New York for an assistant. We directed him to the most convenient cheese stop.

"Thank you again and have a good flight back," I said. Mr. Donahue was met by his driver and we headed toward our car.

"Did you catch that?" asked Terri. "Maybe I misinterpreted it or I'm reading too much into it," she continued, "but he thought that I was the one with MS."

"I agree," I said, "but why do you think so?"

"Just the way he approached me and spoke to me," she said. "He sounded so sympathetic, but I didn't want to embarrass him by saying that you have the MS and not me."

"He meant well and was trying to be supportive," I said. "If I would have been using my cane, he would have thought different. Perhaps, he just got caught in the stereotype about women being three times more likely than men to have MS."

"No," Terri said, "it was like he was saying to me—I'm sorry you have MS." It was a unique opportunity for Terri to experience why I hate sympathetic greetings, and she was clearly upset about being falsely placed in MS shoes. It was an eye-opener for me that even well-informed people can misfire on interpreting MS. The fact was that even though I had MS, I had been no better informed about what it would "look like" for me. Beyond the obvious physical exacerbations that crashed into my life, MS had some invisible and eventful lessons planned for me. It was crucial to realize that MS could simultaneously strike with two distinct fronts of symptoms.

Now imagine there is a disease powerful enough to disrupt nerve connections in the brain, randomly fatiguing and numbing limbs, disrupting balance and equilibrium, and finally, disabling people and disrupting their lives— for many, handing them a cane or a walker or *permanently sitting them into a wheelchair.*

Now imagine that, for most afflicted by this disease, they are surprised by a second silent struggle. These stealth symptoms didn't fit into the box of anticipated physical impediments that was handed to them when their MS was diagnosed. They may be stalled by slowed speed of thinking and recalling their memories. They will be stumped by a delayed recognition of familiar places and faces and keeping up with simple conversations. It is a different kind of numbing, confounding their thoughts and cognitive functions. What was once taken for granted is suddenly unreliable.

Instant access to your thoughts and recalling and articulating information is invisibly stalled; following conversations containing either significant or trivial information becomes muddled and confused; being able to instantly match the correct spoken word with the thought turns into stumbling frustration; the reliable ability to multi-task, absorb interruptions, and remain on the thought track is unexplainably—GONE.

Left with a blank look on their faces, people with MS may feel that they have been seated in an invisible mental wheelchair, just awaiting direction to push their thoughts in the right direction. This is all MS, both the physical and cognitive [thinking] challenges. After living with MS for several years and enduring some initial exacerbations of numbness, loss of vision, and equilibrium, I was stunned by MS disrupting the instant connections in my thinking. Being trapped within my own recollections, but unable to identify or access the information, I was confused about the source of the detachment and terrified of the outcome. Information regarding the cognitive impact of MS for people was scarce and existed only in clinical studies.

Without a clear answer, I was left wondering about my inability to recall my thoughts or recognize familiar locations and faces. It wasn't a topic that I was prepared to either understand or accept on my own. The stigma of mental problems is very real, especially when it is encountered as an imperceptible cognitive bombshell, seemingly unconnected to MS. Denial of the confounded sensation may be normal, but misinformed treatment and ignoring the symptoms should be avoided, since not being able to control your own mind can be terrifying.

The National Multiple Sclerosis Society reports that at least 400,000 people in the U.S. and 2.5 million world-wide have MS. Others believe that the number is much higher, possibly one million in the U.S. alone. Wisconsin has 10,000 people with MS, which means one out of every 500 individuals in the state has MS. Quite frankly, the MS community shouldn't be distracted by these calculations, caught in an endless search for a precise number for the MS population. In any event, the number of people with MS seems to be growing. Whatever the true count, it doesn't change the fact that at least half of people with MS are dealing with varying degrees of cognitive symptoms.

Half!

When you think about MS and that vast group of people, on behalf of them, I ask that you:

- Don't lose sight of the fact that disabilities—whether physical or cognitive—can be equally disabling, disrupting the lives of the affected individuals and their families.
- Don't lose sight of the fact that MS cognitive obstacles and disabilities may be difficult to detect, but are real. "Looking fine" is a cruel illusion.
- Don't lose sight of the fact that, although there is yet no cure for MS, we can slow down progression and enable people to live large and vital lives. When people share examples of how they remain mentally strong and cope with cognitive challenges, their tactical outline is a calm path for others to survive the jams of delayed recall and recognition.

The common themes and strategies by some of the contributing writers to this book are not accidental. In fact, the relevance of their strategies is highlighted by the different ways that the mirrored techniques surface in the lives of individuals who have never met and may live thousands of miles apart from each other. As caring people with MS and medical professionals, the writers share a kindred spirit of tenacity not merely to allow MS cognitive symptoms to exist, but to promote people to reclaim and preserve their cognitive capacity through various avenues of mental exercise and engagement. Their willingness to open very personal moments of encountering and coping with cognitive impediments not only offers validity to the thinking battles endured by numerous people with MS, but is meant to bring the supporting network of friends, family, and medical professionals into the mind of the person. Informed and encouraged by the options to pursue strategies that have been beneficial to others, the writers open options for real hope.

So, reach into the flowing stream of shared cognitive perspectives and strategies, then reach down and scoop up a handful of mental sharpening stones *that work for you.* Use them to stay sharp and hold your cognitive edge against MS.

Acknowledgments

I profoundly appreciate the encouragement and embrace of dear family members and friends—slowly pacing yourselves to assist me on an MS Walk and providing me with the patience and mental running room to complete thoughts and commitments, you keep me physically and cognitively motivated and connected with true purpose.

For Noreen Henson and Richard Johnson of Demos Medical Publishing. Nicole Fletcher and Biogen Idec, Inc., EMD Serono, and Teva Neuroscience—thank you for your tremendous support for this project of bringing successful strategies for dealing with MS cognitive difficulties into an open and accessible discussion for people with MS, their families, and the medical professionals who care for them.

Also, thank you to my fellow speedskaters, Bruce Conner, Marv Hughes, Bob Fenn, and Bonnie Blair—for setting the standard of physical conditioning and mental focus, while maintaining your sharp edges. For Chris Zapf, who helped me to maintain the clear accuracy of shared cognitive conversations and for Peggy Morsch, who captures me in crisp light.

Thank you to all medical professionals like Drs. Maas and Matthais, who, because of your comprehensive understanding of both the cognitive and physical aspects of MS, recognize that opening the MS cognitive discussion is vital to treating people's difficulties and promoting their quality of life. And to all therapists who help collect the various MS puzzle pieces and assist those people with MS to assemble a functional picture for themselves.

I am grateful to the President of the *National Multiple Sclerosis Society*, Joyce Nelson, and especially the Wisconsin Chapter and its President, Colleen Kalt, along with Mary Hartwig, Bonnie DeBroux, Erica Hartsough, Jeremy Otte, and Amy Reinicke for passionately reaching out to the MS community and for providing the consistent energy and support for everyone involved in the effort to advocate, educate, and support research to improve treatments for MS. From the *National MS Society*, to the *Montel Williams MS Foundation*, the *Rocky Mountain MS Center*, and the *MS Foundation*, we are united arm-in-arm with sister organizations around the world like the *MS Society* and *Multiple Sclerosis Resource Centre* in the UK, who all recognize and insist on informed, compassionate, and accessible care for people with MS.

A special thanks to the all of the individuals who have contributed their outstanding honest writing and discussion to this book. These people reflect the best efforts of the MS community at-large, providing us with real hope for better understanding and treatment, ultimately moving us closer to a cure for MS.

Mental Sharpening Stones

CHAPTER 1

Sharpening Conversations

Jeffrey N. Gingold

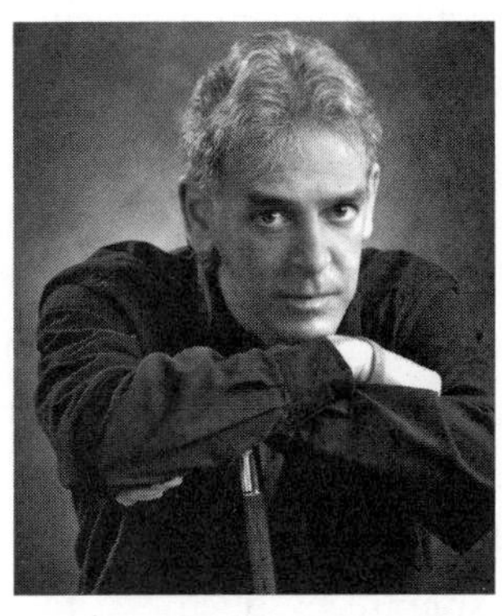

Jeffrey N. Gingold, enjoying a calm moment at his home on the East side of Milwaukee, pondering speedskating. Photo © Peggy Morsch.

"Do you have a group photo with everyone from the book?" At the time of this book's release, most of the individuals who have contributed their personal insight to this MS cognitive discussion have not met each other. However, their approaches to MS hold common threads. It was a quiet tapestry of individuals who have discovered their resiliency to preclude and cope with their private curveballs of MS cognitive symptoms—without acquiescing.

This first chapter reveals this striking theme. Whether producing cutting-edge journalism, succeeding as an Emmy Award winning television Talk Show Host or administering to an entire state judicial system, these conversations convey their parallel approaches. Avoiding the cognitive challenges of MS through disuse and isolation of the mind were never options.

These three people display a keen sense of humanity, sharing their passion and learned expertise of how to excel, even when mentally or physically side-swiped by MS. Their stories are personal invitations to prepare, understand and move on.

Coping Without Yielding

A Conversation with Richard Cohen

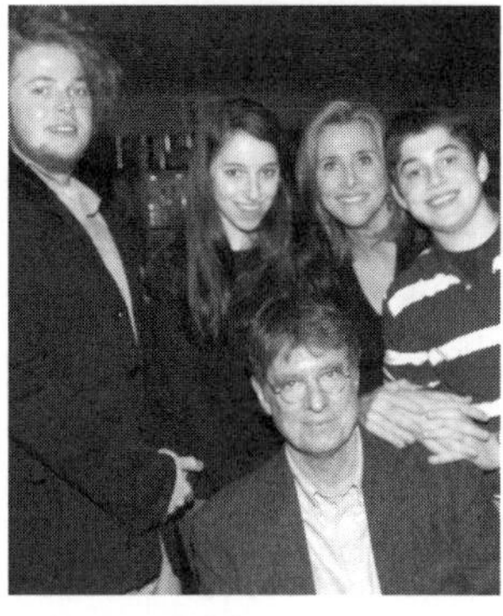

Richard Cohen is a three-time Emmy and John Foster Peabody award-winning, network television news producer and a New York Times *best-selling author. Acknowledging and learning to understand the cognitive aspects of MS, Richard has discovered how to calmly pace himself through perplexing moments without surrendering either his work or enjoyment of life.*

After returning home from a late Friday night dinner at our favorite Italian restaurant, my wife, Terri, suggested that I listen to the message on the answering machine. When I tried to wave off the message until the morning, she insisted that I would want to listen to it now and write down the details myself. It wasn't a telephone call that I had expected, and the honesty of the message was engaging.

"My name is Richard Cohen," the message began. "I live in New York and I have MS. I was told about your [MS cognitive book] project and I am more than happy to talk to you about it." There was a few seconds of silence. "What's my number?" he said, sounding a bit exasperated. "I guess that makes the point!" Cohen laughed. He paused again and then left his phone number, asking that I call him.

There were actually two messages within the one blinking light on our answering machine. The first was that Cohen was interested in the multiple sclerosis (MS) cognitive topic of this book and, the second, that he would be willing to share his very personal MS cognitive challenges. His numerous awards for journalism, including three *Emmys* and a *John Foster Peabody*, were illustrative of his ability to investigate and convey the salient points of critical issues and personalities. His manner of providing honest insight could also turn on a light in the closet of invisible MS symptoms.

Paid Dues

Cohen is not a new figure in the public health discussion. He is a contributor to the health and fitness pages of *The New York Times* and author of *Blindsided: Lifting a Life above Illness* (2004), a *New York Times* bestseller. In *Blindsided*, Cohen discusses how he was struck by two life-stunning diseases and had to acknowledge the changes forced upon him without losing his sense of purpose for a successful family and journalism career.

When he was diagnosed with MS in 1973, he was an associate producer with *ABC News*, covering the Watergate hearings. He subsequently worked with *The MacNeil/Lehrer Report* on public television, as a producer on the *CBS Evening News with Walter Cronkite*, and then as Dan Rather's producer when Rather moved to the anchor position in 1981.

"Cohen says he never turned down an assignment, no matter how stressful or dangerous," noted an article in the July/August 2007 issue of *Neurology Today*. When Cohen was with CBS News, he reported on the rise of the Solidarity trade-union movement in Poland and on wars in the Middle East and Central America. He later managed the CBS News coverage of the 1984 and 1988 presidential campaigns and traveled with President Reagan to China in 1984.

Cohen returned to PBS in 1989, joining Bill Moyers to produce and direct *Illusions of News*, an award-winning documentary about the press. In 1992, he joined CNN, covering the election of Bill Clinton and producing another award-winning documentary entitled, *Bill Clinton of Arkansas*. Although MS traveled with Cohen on all assignments, there seemed to be no suggestion of him slowing down. On the contrary, his determination seems to have been fueled by any hint that he no longer should pursue his work.

Although MS was a private reality for Cohen and his family, the disease needed to move aside for a more pressing concern. As if dealing with the exacerbations and disability from MS would not be enough, in 1999 Cohen was diagnosed and treated for colon cancer. He found himself facing the cruel and humbling disease again within another year. Cohen had never set out to prove how strong he was or how determined a person could be when faced with life-slamming confrontations, twice, but he would not let MS or the double round of cancer sidetrack his vision of a having both a successful family and a successful career. Although denial may not be one of the FDA-approved medications to deal with either disease, Cohen's ability to provide a healthy self-administered dose of denial has given him the fortitude and vision to challenge the diseases, share his story, and educate others, possibly beyond his own initial expectations.

By personally defining his existence, despite the life tremors, Richard Cohen demonstrates a subtle smile of resistance. He deflects the true impact of MS brain lesions, just like some people can firmly say "no thank-you" to an unsolicited door-to-door salesperson. Cohen has too much yet to accomplish to be slowed down by self-pity or MS detours. With a discernable and provocative bend toward taking his physical and cognitive challenges head on, without any hint of self-destruction, Cohen has set his sights on what he wants to accomplish. With rich purpose, life is very good.

Cohen's attitude is exemplified by the title of his book that he was writing at the time of our early conversations: *Strong at the Broken Places: Voices of Illness, a Chorus of Hope* (HarperCollins, 2008). The stories that he shares reflect the core strength of individuals who face otherwise catastrophic health conditions. By facing down his own personal health struggles, Cohen gained the profound understanding and connection to those individuals whose strength is revealed in the book. The positive ripple effects from those shared stories will be felt in countless families, initiating their own unseen ripples.

Providing beneficial information has been a common theme throughout Cohen's reporting career. However, as he pursued investigative work and produced documentaries that deeply probed meaningful subjects and powerful individuals, Cohen was unaware of how MS was slowly infiltrating his body and would ultimately influence his life beyond the understood physical obstacles that are faced by people with MS.

The Unknown MS

At the time of the Watergate hearings, Cohen's personal life was about to turn upside down. Unlike members of the Nixon administration, who probably could have foreseen the likely outcome of their conduct, Cohen had no hint of what was waiting for him. No one had mentioned the stealth cognitive hurdles that were lurking in his MS diagnosis.

"It was weird," said Cohen, thinking about the time that he was working for *ABC News*. "Some days I was in the hearing and other days in the tape room." It was an action that he may have unconsciously done countless times, but, on this one day, the simple task of placing tapes in their containers was confounding. "What really threw me was that it was a conceptual confusion," Cohen explained. Years before the use of CDs, DVDs, and other digital formats, recordings were made on reel-to-reel tapes. They could be unwieldy to deal with, especially when the tapes jammed or the receiving reel did not wrap the tape, depositing it on the floor as a heap of shiny ribbon.

"It was different from the minor confusion that normal people, especially a 25-year-old, would have," recalled Cohen. "It was the tape setting, how you fit it around and into a round container. It was weird. You had to put it in a certain way and I had done it a thousand times and suddenly, I was confused about it." The frustration wasn't worth explaining to anyone, and Cohen may have simply assumed that he was exhausted by the hearings and needed more rest. Based upon his early understanding of the disease, Cohen didn't attribute the confusion to MS. Perhaps similar to other relapsing-remitting MS symptoms, this incident came and went without any alarm sounded by Cohen.

"The truth of the matter is that the recognition of cognitive problems really came after a while," noted Cohen. "It didn't come at the beginning. I was totally oblivious to everything and much more focused on the purely physical." This is not unusual, since most of the patient literature, especially at the time of Cohen's diagnosis, emphasizes the physical symptoms. The cognitive interference from MS was outside of the box of symptoms that were described to patients and their families. Without having any causal link between cognitive issues and MS, Cohen didn't mention the incident to anyone, not even his doctor.

"I certainly wasn't going to tell any of the people I worked with about it. A lot of times, cognitive problems are larger in our heads than it would be in anybody else's," explained Cohen. "I know that cognitive problems that I see on a regular basis are never noticed by anybody else. I had noticed them clearly in speaking engagements in which my neurologist was in the audience, and he didn't notice it."

A person using a cane is easy to identify as dealing with a disability, but it is difficult for others to notice when an individual's recall is slowed. Although it can be obvious to appreciate that a person with a walker will have difficulty maneuvering down the stairs, the inability to find the right words or memory is not easily detected. The sensation of losing your thoughts or being unable to accomplish what was previously a "no-brainer" can leave a person temporarily bewildered, whether it is a serious or trivial moment.

Perhaps similar to experiencing a "senior" moment, an MS cognitive moment can temporarily shut down people with MS, leaving them wondering about what just happened or why a routine task is now perplexing. Trying to articulate the phenomenon to a family member, friend, or physician may be daunting, trying to explain the unexplainable. Surrounding the unknown symptoms with silence leaves people with MS in a mental wheelchair. The obstruction is invisible, even to a medical professional, and often not completely understood by the individual dealing with the moment.

When Cohen is aware of the cognitive delay in his thoughts, it is silently frustrating for him to lose a thought. "It's like a drop-off," said Cohen. "You just reach for words, and you know what you want to say, but you can't find the word to say it." Although he may find no easy escape from the words being snatched away, Cohen understands how to not make the moment worse and perhaps noticeable to others, while struggling to articulate what had been on the tip of tongue.

"You reach a little further and you calm yourself for a second, and it seems like an eternity," Cohen paused, possibly recalling public moments of uncomfortable self-recognition. "It seems like an eternity and the fact is, in public speaking, there are plenty of pauses, and nobody thinks it's significant." The good news is that no one else may notice that MS-weighted thoughts are resting on mental quicksand and quickly vanish beneath the present moment. Rapid digging for a sinking thought seems to only push it further down while more layers of distracting information bits pile on top.

Cohen had spoken to the American Academy of Neurology at its annual meeting and had some difficulties with the hour-long presentation. "I have real trouble when I speak because my eyes are so bad. I don't look at anything," said Cohen. "I could never read a speech, so what I have to do is organize my mind." Since presenting a speech may be tough for anyone, Cohen understands that he needs to cut himself extra slack to get through the presentations. When you cannot refer to a written speech or notes, having your thoughts organized in a reachable manner is vital to covering the topic.

Personally, I have often wished that someone in the "wings" would toss me a line when MS vacates my thoughts, but no one else can know what I have just forgotten. True and accurate mind-readers are rare. Even Cohen's wife, Meredith Vieira, may not be able to find the words for him. As a host on The Today Show, Vieira certainly knows her way around an interview or conversation. She can sense when Cohen is having trouble finding the words and would like to alleviate his frustration. However, there is no instant solution to pulling out the correct words.

"She gets very impatient," noted Cohen. "It's like she's motioning, come on, come on. I always say, 'Meredith, this is not a talk-show, this is real life.'" Cohen appreciates that his wife is trying to help with his moments of cognitive delay. He also understands that it is natural for her to offer assistance when he is groping for words or a lost thought and trying to connect it with the correct spoken phrase. What seems clear is that neither party can force the recall of the stray thought.

"You can't stick the words in their mouths," said Cohen, "but I think what people do too often is allow themselves to get agitated." Whether a person is getting irritated with himself or with the individual suggesting words and trying to move the thought along, it can be a slippery slope of mental exasperation. "Once you start getting agitated, it's going to be harder to find the words." Cohen's solution is practical and, with a little calm self-assurance, it can be learned by many others who may experience the same unpredictable diversions in their conversations.

"I have learned to switch gears a little bit," said Cohen, "just angle it a little bit, and then I can usually find my way back pretty easily." Backing away from the confused or lost thought is not necessarily giving up the point but, rather, relieving the pressure on the bottleneck of thoughts with patience and allowing the bottleneck to unclog itself. Cohen's suggestion took me back to my teenage attempts to parallel park my father's 1966 fire-engine red Ford Galaxie 500. At age 16, I had received my driver's license and was assumed to suddenly possess the skill to park a Sherman tank in the empty space between any two curbside-parked cars.

Attempting to back the Goliath-size car into a curb space from a bad angle could never be improved with increased speed or by sharply spinning the steering wheel in any direction. There is a blunt honesty from the sound of clunking bumpers, combined with a distinct jolting sensation. I could either remain trapped by the awkward position or "switch gears" and pull out of the pinned-in situation. When I have lost my words and feel pinned by a conversation that I suddenly can't follow, the stuck sensation is similar the feeling that occurs with a bad parallel-parking job with the front of the car precariously sticking out in the traffic lane. Cohen's strategy: keep calm and gracefully pull away from the jammed moment, then try it again later from a different angle.

The strategy asks one to admit that whatever you were doing wasn't working and to face the fact that you may need to back out and start over. This doesn't mean leaving the building where the conversation is taking place. As Cohen suggests, you leave just enough room to come at it again from a slightly different angle. If you pull too far away, then the mental parking place and the conversation may be gone. Cohen recommends a second strategy to retrieve the lost track of thought. "Just be patient," he continued, "just don't react by filling in the gaps." Tossing in random guesses may only further distract your mind from the original missing word or idea. A support person can be equally frustrated by the stagnant conversation and, despite their best intentions, they can derail a calm approach to getting back on track by overcompensating with too much information.

"Meredith does that to me," said Cohen. "Meredith will already start guessing answers. I say—when you're done guessing the answer . . . I think that the temptation to play the game is much greater when you're sensing someone is really grasping or groping for something." Once others allow the mental running room for the individual to relax and be patient, the words tend to return by pursuing a different direction on the topic. For a support person, silent assistance may seem empty of substance. However, protecting the individual's cognitive space and allowing him to calmly switch thinking gears may provide the greatest probability to connect with the words or concepts that have seemingly vanished.

Catching the Details

Getting mentally "lost" may not be limited to verbal skills and may also include other mental processes, such as following instructions, whether simple or detailed. For Cohen, he has found that even dealing with simple tasks and following directions has become more challenging. It is one matter to read instructions and quite another to have the absorbed detail translated into the use of words or hands. Many people without MS would state that they have that type of difficulty, but for those individuals with MS, it may reflect a more classic cognitive disconnection.

"The most noticeable thing to me is that I have a total loss of memory for people's names," said Cohen. His awareness extends beyond merely not remembering the names of recently introduced faces. "I can be in a group of people I know well, and if I had to introduce them to each other, I would have difficulty doing it." Second guessing what you think you should know can be petrifying and humbling. "I always live in fear of being with somebody and having to introduce him or her to somebody else," said Cohen. Instead of recoiling at the thought of embarrassment, Cohen's voice held the reverberation of resolve to not avoid anything.

When I shared with him that I too am regularly at a loss to recall a name or a face, even the ones that are close to me, we discovered that we shared a cognitive strategy. When my wife and I run into friends and relatives, she can assume that I will not remember their names and so, I will introduce her first with "you remember my wife, Terri." When she extends her hand, the person will respond to her and offer their name. If it turns out that it is an individual that I should have known, which often occurs, then we all laugh at the formal-sounding comment and leave it there.

"That's so funny because I do that to Meredith or a friend," said Cohen. When he is alone, recognition becomes more complicated because of his vision loss. "I'm legally blind, so I don't see faces well enough to remember them sometimes." It is a double challenge, since clearly seeing a face and recalling a name may both be compromised. The problematic encounter can be further compounded if Cohen receives information from the individual. "Another way the problem presents itself is that a person I know well can give me a piece of complicated information," continued Cohen. "I will digest that information, go home, remember the information in perfect detail, and have no idea who told it—no idea." The experience was as common and recent for Cohen as the day before our last conversation.

As a result of Cohen's journalism background, he is always keeping up with people in the news and in tune with political coverage. "I'm always talking politics with people, so in a given day, I could talk to anywhere from a half dozen to 10 people," noted Cohen. "There's always information. I get more gossip than could ever be on television and news, but I can't remember who told me." Cohen acknowledges the interruptions in his information processing and that "it's such a clear pattern that it's a liability." Understanding the difficulty is not the end game for Cohen but, instead, the first step to accepting responsibility for the roadblocks on the path to his goals. "It's very hard to know whether I'm having difficulty due to aging, to MS, or to too many good times in the 60s," said Cohen. "It's hard to know what to attribute the difficulties to, but there are certain things that are very clearly MS."

At times, MS may seem like a deceiving annoyance to Cohen, but without allowing himself to freak out, he is able to assess the mental change-up and then get back on the right mental track. "A couple of times I have taken the subway and when we switch lines, I find myself up on the street, and I have thought to myself, why did I do that, I was just switching trains?" Fortunately, Cohen knows the subway system and quickly realizes when he has made an exit mistake. With humility in check, it only costs Cohen the price of a ticket to re-enter the subway turnstile. Until a person has experienced a moment of location bafflement, it may be difficult to comprehend the shock and instant frustration associated with an unanticipated scenery change. When MS has played bait and switch with your taken-for-granted reality, a calm acknowledgement of the occurrence may be the best strategy to deal with the temporary disorientation.

Just imagine becoming lost near your own neighborhood. Perhaps you walk into a room in your house and pause, unable to understand why you went there. Wouldn't it be a startling moment to discover that you just sat down at a neighbor's kitchen table for dinner, thinking that you were at home? Now you have to back yourself away from the wrong place setting and go home. The awkwardness may only be internal, as the uninvited guest, but you still have to wonder why you appeared there and now need to find the least dramatic way to return back to the intended table, sharing the chair with MS.

Cohen knows the New York subway and with that upbringing in his mental history, he understands how to acknowledge the moments of bafflement and safely wait out the misdirection. He appreciates that the cognitive turmoil may surface at will. Despite grappling with MS impediments, Cohen has come to terms with the disease and is determined to focus on what he can accomplish, moving beyond any mental sidesteps.

"I would be going to Grand Central Station and Times Square on the shuttle, and go up Broadway to my studio apartment and I find myself standing on 42nd and Broadway and saying—why am I up here? Why did I do that?" wondered Cohen. "I go upstairs in my house and I don't have a clue why I walked upstairs." Cohen appears to have found some comfort in following an analytical path through these disquieting moments of his *loss of presence.*

Contemplating the eccentricities of the brain on a personal level, he realized that it is occurring to him on more than an occasional basis. He may find himself trying to make sense out of articles of clothing and wondering what goes where. "Do you put your legs through a sweater?" Cohen would contemplate. "It's a momentary thing and I'm stuck, but I think it through." The uncanny visual image is acknowledged by Cohen as an unusual course in the brain, and then it is calmly put aside without distraction from known reality. Perhaps one of the most disturbing facets of walking into slight cognitive shifts is the unpredictability of the perplexing thought. What was once an unconscious routine may suddenly become a fixated point of a unique puzzlement.

"I was standing in the shower area at the gym" noted Cohen, "and went to toss my shorts onto a rack on the wall at shoulder height. I could not figure out how to do it and started and stopped a few times and tossed them onto a bench a foot away instead. I then repeated the move and completed this complicated task immediately. Scary." What might have been more unsettling to Cohen would have been to allow himself to melt down at the stone-walling encounter with the gym rack. However, he was prepared for such bizarre moments of cognitive delay and had a plan in place to pace his way through the episode.

Although approximately half of the MS population may face some level of cognitive impairment, the manner and timing of the interference with the mind can vary from person to person and day to day. There may be some common themes that most people with MS will encounter, whether through the moments of diagnosis, treatment, and personal adaptation. The physical and cognitive symptoms and disabilities that I deal with as a person living with MS may have great similarity with Cohen's experiences, but our individual events are associated with our specific environments and do not mirror a future course of challenges.

The same may be said for any roomful of people with MS. They may head-nod on their initial symptoms that brought them to diagnosis and the neurologist's recommendation for choice of medication, but from there, the personal experience may be modified by age, overall health, current family structure, employment and quality of health insurance—the list goes on. However, although the details of an MS experience may be individualized, the use of another person's strategies saves others from having to create the MS wheel of coping techniques for themselves. Richard Cohen's stirring fight for maintaining his vitality is not only inspiring, but an open invitation to other people with MS to share their stories of coping with cognitive disconnection.

A Calm Approach

Facing the truth about the cognitive aspects of MS and acting with patience for himself, Cohen has employed simple, yet powerfully effective strategies to manage the disturbing mental jumble. One of Cohen's most important and consistent responses to instances of cognitive quicksand is to immediately shift his focus to calming down his mind and relaxing the speed of his thoughts. The quieting effect of this practice allows him to observe the confounded moment as just another fleeting incident. The information is not lost, but obscured, which may delay instant recall or recognition.

"Whatever it is, it comes back," notes Cohen. "I will tell you that there's stuff that could take hours to come back to, like who said what today, but the rest of it's resolved relatively quickly." When he gave a speech for approximately 300 doctors, Cohen wondered whether they would notice anything regarding his cognitive blank moments. They apparently did not. "Any number of them, I would have thought, would have caught the problems, and nobody saw anything." With a calm approach to encountering MS cognitive meddling, Cohen moves forward with the confidence that the information will surface, avoiding the added pressure of demanding instant recall.

For Cohen, it is important "to relax and to accept the two seconds of silence or, if you think it's not going to be acceptable, to sort of pray a little bit and then come back to that." A person may not be able to force or predict the return of a disconnected thought, but there seems to be a better opportunity for recovery if you keep your thoughts moving. "The bridge is successfully crossed much more quickly than we think it is," said Cohen. Let it go and keep the thoughts flowing along.

Cohen's appreciation of MS cognitive roadblocks reminded me of our recent family trip to the Black Hills of South Dakota. While driving through and around edgy cliffs, we would see signs stating: "Beware of Falling Rocks." The signs didn't say "Go Back" or "Freak Out and Be Frightened." The message instilled us with awareness as we moved forward with the traveling adventure past sculpted mountain portraits. Even if we were compelled to stop, we would back up and go in a different direction toward the destination. If Cohen would forget the next comment that he was going to state, then he might find another point to review and patiently wait for the misplaced thought to emerge again through another direction.

By avoiding a specific message track or being bound to fixed wording, Cohen is better able to connect his thoughts for a presentation. Because of his bad eyesight, Cohen has learned to conceptualize his speaking points, writing down a couple of notes as preparation, but not for word-to-word reference during a speech. For him, it is a matter of discipline to prepare from a couple of notes and self-control to continue thinking through the message, keeping a structure in his head. In a way, Cohen works off of the "PowerPoint" in his mind and doesn't need a computer projector. If Cohen was offered the use of a plugged-in PowerPoint presentation, he noted that it was an unnecessary crutch and a barrier to a personal connection to people.

To keep his mind active on a different level, Cohen maintains his interest by listening to a broad range of music. He especially enjoys attending the opera and classical music concerts, finding it very calming. Although his wife's work schedule may be demanding and tends to operate on an opposite time zone, Cohen is comfortable pursuing concerts on his own. "Meredith, because she is a hostess of *The Today Show*, gets up at 3:00 in the morning and works in the evenings, so she's a lost soul," noted Cohen. "So I'm just going to do this kind of stuff by myself."

He prefers to immerse himself in the music that seems to exercise his mind. "I find classical music to be very evocative; it's a part of memory to me that I have a lot of association with over the years. The calming effect of the music is never white noise for Cohen and instead, provides a basis for using his analytical skills to key in on specific instruments and movements, following the intricacies of the performance. It is possible to better appreciate the draw of a specific piece of music by allowing the brain to pick up on the countless elements that contribute to the sound. The satisfaction of deeply absorbing classical music allows Cohen to pleasantly examine the complexities of the composition, providing mental exertion on the level of cognitive calisthenics.

Such a mental aerobic workout may pay dividends as Cohen sorts through and assembles the chapters of his new book, *Strong at the Broken Places: Voices of Illness, a Chorus of Hope*. The book profiles five people from all over the country, living with chronic illnesses. Sorting through the influx of information from interviews, assembling notes, and drafting chapters was manageable for Cohen, primarily because he set the expectations and timing for himself. Although he may not find the cognitive delays to be an issue when writing, the obstruction may rear its head at simple moments.

"I also have developed a disconnect for the spelling of routine words. I write them and doubt they are spelled correctly," noted Cohen. "Generally they are, but they do not look correct." He relies on a freelance editor to also work on the book project, which allows him to talk through interesting points. This was a successful process that he also utilized for writing *Blindsided*.

Cohen understands that the best way to minimize any interference from the "cognitive stuff" is to work within his own space, "without time pressures and nobody looking at me," said Cohen.

"When you're writing a book," said Cohen, "you're writing at your own pace. There's no performance in that." By setting his own writing schedule, he avoided interference from cognitive delays and loss of information. With that bit of control, "my challenges were much more sight oriented with a ton of transcripts to go through." Cohen has identified his best window of time for writing, remaining mindful about not wasting the opportunity when energy and his mental focus are sharp.

"I decline throughout the day," said Cohen. "I'm at my best as soon as I wake up." Fatigue may be one of the most common complaints from people with MS, and Cohen noticed that, "if I don't have my best energy in the morning, it's a bad day." With that appreciation for the working margins of MS, Cohen is not deterred from meeting his own expectations. Some may say that is classic denial, to insist on struggling through work. Those who may understand this balance of enduring an MS drag, while in pursuit of "normal" physical and cognitive days, are actually witnessing Cohen's sheer determination and nothing less.

"I think that we're prisoners of the world," explained Cohen. "The world isn't going to slow down for us. If you're a clerk in a store, people are throwing things at you. If you're a pharmacist, people are ordering things, and you're going to have to make peace with it." And when you are limited by MS and cannot work more efficiently to meet the expectations thrust upon you, then the best options may be to adjust the preset targets and modes of function—both appropriate strategies. Knowing the difference between pre-MS demand levels with a new adjusted set of expectations may be crucial to avoid setting yourself up for failure.

"I just think that the best thing you can do, when you have the luxury of doing it," noted Cohen, "is slowing down, staying calm, and buying yourself a little bit of time." Being patient with yourself and very realistic about any new cognitive stumbling blocks may, in fact, allow you to either catch up or duck and avoid being struck by the items tossed at you. Doing so may also lead you to a productive place where you will also find some peace.

Pure Resolve

Maybe MS wasn't the disease that Cohen had first thought it would be for him, and it took a while for him to come to grips with the "progressive" part of having a progressive disease. "I think a lot of us play the game," explained Cohen, "I accept it for what it is now. Lord knows its wreaked havoc on me, but let's just say—I will accept it and it won't get worse. That's the bargain you want to make to nobody in particular, and obviously it doesn't work that way." With that understanding about MS, Cohen remains realistic about the cognitive aspects of a progressive disease.

This may be especially true for Cohen who considers himself to be a creature of the mind, more than the body. "I think it would be particularly devastating to see that happening to myself," said Cohen, but he won't allow himself to go there. And with that dose of healthy denial in place, he lives focused on the temporary nature of the random cognitive change-up in his thoughts and not on whether the frequency or intensity might progress.

Perhaps like a soccer goalie defending against a team of MS, each player simultaneously firing soccer balls at him from different directions, Cohen knows not to remain still and allow easy points to be scored against him. When describing how he further challenges his mind, beyond various writing endeavors, his answer is simple. "I read," said Cohen, "I mean, I read!" Since he is legally blind, he has trouble reading and uses very powerful glasses with prisms in the middle. "They're magnifiers, so I have to hold the book very close to my eyes." Cohen's physical impediments from MS may be obstacles, but they are not barriers to him.

"I have a bad habit of buying long books," said Cohen, as he explained that he just bought a 750-page book. "It's too heavy to carry anywhere and I almost don't have the strength in my arms right now." That might be an obstacle for some people. "My right arm is too bad to hold it up to read it, so I have to rest it on the arm of the chair and then lunge over to read it." That is a definition of bounding over a barrier—by Cohen. In pursuit of remaining cognitively connected, he concedes that nothing is easy. "You do what you can do as long as you can do it," Cohen asserted. Even when it may surprise others, he will continue to live large and as functional as possible.

"When *Blindsided* came out, we did this big thing with Barbara Walters, and she couldn't get over the fact that I still take the subway." Walters asked him why he still did that. "And my answer is, because I can," said Cohen. "You see, because that's who I am, and I'm going to read 750-page books until I can't do it anymore." Cohen's determination to challenge his mind in the face of startling recognition shifts is exemplified by his resolve to read until he can't hold the weighty book or focus on the magnified print. "I guess my own stubborn strength has surprised me," admitted Cohen. Harnessed denial can be a powerful companion.

Cohen has witnessed the MS cognitive drag on his reporting skills, but with adjustments in his information gathering, he is able to pursue the contacts and the story. The opportunity to receive information will not be missed by Cohen, and the modified methods may be imperceptible to others.

"Numbers and handwriting get me, and taking messages is impossible," said Cohen. "I tell the truth and ask people to e-mail numbers whenever possible." The honest request enables him to receive accurate information without concern for missing out on vital details. "Looking at numbers—what I have scrawled on a check or paying for a credit card purchase—is harder than it used to be. The numbers do not make immediate sense." Acknowledging the delayed numbers' connection is a crucial step toward not making mistakes, when combined with a repetition method for verification. The thought of no longer writing is not contemplated by Cohen, especially since he can find other methods to do his work. The same philosophy applies to his exercise routine, which provides both physical and cognitive benefits to him.

"That's a good thing, you know," said Cohen, "that I can go to the gym in the morning. I can't do what I used to do, but I still do what I can do." It is a successful approach: don't stop cognitive and physical challenges, even in the face of diminished results. That may be the most underestimated strategy of all. If you stop completely, even when the routine becomes more difficult, then there will be no benefit whatsoever. A mind or muscle doesn't get exercised by stillness.

In addition to the direct physical benefits from exercising, Cohen also feels that there is a connection to being able to maintain his cognitive sharpness. "Feeling like you're holding onto some control with an illness, where there's very little control, calms the mind," noted Cohen. As a well-traveled journalist, Cohen acknowledges that his career has taken him around the world, into war zones, and face-to-face with political and social turmoil. Transferring those encounters into meaningful stories that bring readers into the very moment of discussion may feed Cohen's thoughts, which are constantly churning through concepts and interviews.

"I have an uncalm mind," said Cohen. "I have a restless mind to begin with, and I think that's exacerbated by the illness. And to whatever degree I can genuinely feel that I'm holding onto some control, having no illusions, it keeps other problems at a minimum and I think it's calming." Exercising his body to help calm himself enables his mind to settle down and cognitively process the overwhelming incoming information.

"I do some aerobic exercising," said Cohen. "I have a bad knee and a weak leg because of the MS, and that makes it difficult." As opposed to skipping out on the routine and instead, crashing down into a cushy chair at home, Cohen is not deterred from the effort. "I am able to work on that and do a little bit of weights. Compared to what I used to do, it's pathetic, but I think there's a real psychological pay off for continuing to do what you want to do, what you think you can do." His exercises are linked to the determination of wanting to be physically active and to remaining calm and cognitively vibrant to continue writing. By Cohen's definition, it is never worth saying that it isn't worth it anymore. Using diminishing returns for exercise as an excuse to quit working out may have a domino effect, later impeding his thinking processes. There is too much at stake to skip staying fit.

While absorbing the relentless streams of information, enjoying family time, and being pinched between colon cancer and MS, Cohen accepts that life can be extremely stressful. He has told many people that, given a choice between ridding himself of the side-effects from two rounds of colon cancer or MS, he would choose the colon cancer.

"I have had it twice," said Cohen, "and having the surgery and losing parts of my intestines, digestion, and all that stuff is not a picnic. It's a daily problem." With that blunt perspective, Cohen cannot identify with those who allow themselves to remain trapped in a self-pity mode. "That's unacceptable, and if you choose to be a professional victim, then you have to go with what you've got and make it work." Despite having to endure being blasted by the double barrels of life-altering health traumas, Cohen will not be relegated to a role of incapable patient. His wife, Meredith, has received random phone calls from people with a sympathetic twang wanting to know "*How is Richard?*" Cohen's reaction to the overly sympathetic tone is in line with—pleeeasse, you have got to be kidding.

When familiar faces and locations are temporarily obscured and information becomes more difficult to absorb or recall, Cohen has figured out how to cope without being caught in the pity trap. Whether it is the adapted exercise routine, the mentally stimulating conversations and performances, or sheer independence of movement with a calm self-discipline, it all works for him. Cohen trusts himself to know that offering him a mournful hand doesn't help and instead, might slow him down. Since he won't give up on himself, no one should expect otherwise from him or perhaps—themselves.

"The fact of the matter is, I have an exciting life," said Cohen. "I have had a life of doing different things, to really do what I wanted to do, and I have got a great family." And for Cohen, it is not merely a convenient outlook of how his life has evolved. "That's the only perspective as far as I'm concerned," said Cohen, with the resolve of not only knowing where he has been, but embracing where he will go. There is a difference between being a career victim and a relentless survivor.

With honesty and perseverance, Cohen is the latter and he has the credentials to prove it.

Mental Sharpening Stones and Perspectives

1. When faced with moments of delayed recognition and slowed thoughts, realize that it is temporary and relax. The missing thought or lost presence will come back to you.
2. If it is difficult to absorb information and accurately record it, then ask others to back-up useful information by writing it down for you or e-mailing the details for later reference.
3. Define your existence by learning to pace out thinking impediments, and continuing to pursue your abilities with adaptive techniques.
4. Attend performances that calm your mind and stimulate your thoughts by observing the nuances of the production. Seek out delightful mental exertion.

5. Define your best functioning pace, and set deadlines within those flexible boundaries.
6. Reduce your exposure to "toxic" overly sympathetic conversation. Relish your abilities and work to your edge of physical exercise and mental challenges.
7. Determination is born from being told by others that you no longer should or can, then figuring how to accomplish it. To whatever level you are able to do something, continue to do it.

Leading by Open Example

A Conversation with Montel Williams

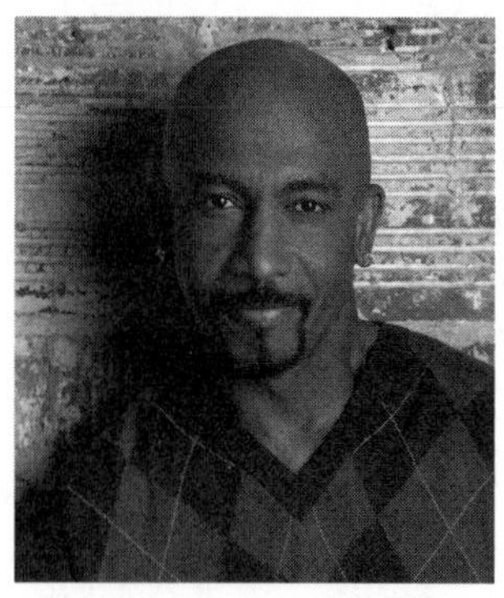

Montel Williams is a national television talk-show host, a New York Times *best-selling author, and founder of* The Montel Williams MS Foundation. *Montel discusses how welcoming new mental challenges may foster cognitive endurance and growth of the mind.*

"Would you come to New York to be on the show with Montel?" asked Stacey, one of the producers for *The Montel Williams Show*. "He would like to meet you and discuss your book about cognitive MS symptoms." Caught frozen like a deer in the headlights of an oncoming truck, I was stunned by the question and quickly glanced at the caller ID. Discovering the New York City telephone number on the screen, I snapped out of my trance and quickly agreed to the request.

My first book, *Facing the Cognitive Challenges of Multiple Sclerosis*, had only been released a few weeks earlier, and although I was pleased with the very kind and enthusiastic book reviews, I hadn't thought about national television interviews, much less the undesired stress on my MS symptoms. The next week, a camera crew was at our home to film candid interviews with me, my wife, Terri, and our girls, Lauren and Meredith. The questions were blunt, while the straight answers were emotionally revealing and draining for all of us. After five hours of taped conversations and re-enactments, I was physically fatigued, hobbled by my partially numb left leg and tilted equilibrium, but those weren't the only MS hits to my body. When the taping was finished, I sat on the couch, mentally fried and unable to clearly string two thoughts together. My day was sliced short. As my body began to tremor and my legs buckled, Terri held my arm as I gingerly climbed the stairs.

"Will you be up for eating a bit later?" asked Terri. Perhaps sensing that my thoughts were also frayed, she understood the head shake "no." MS landed me in bed before 8:00 p.m. on a weekend night. Although the film crew's computers, cameras, and flood and spot lights hadn't blown a fuse in our home, the heat from the lighting and interview stress had tripped my MS-loaded nerve connections. When Terri asked me the next day about my interview answers, I was stumped and blank. It was unnerving not being able to recall what I might have said on camera, but I trusted Montel's editors to use the coherent statements or piece them together.

It was a draining interview about my book dealing with the first-person impact from MS cognitive impediments—and my brain shut down. This is one of the reasons that I was compelled to retire as an attorney. I was unsure about what was asked and how I responded; MS is a constant lesson about my limits of recall and thinking fatigue. The irony of the interview topic and result was obvious as I began to wonder about the potential fallout from the New York trip.

There was no cause to stress about preparing for the show. Self-inflicted stress serves no purpose other than to further exacerbate my MS symptoms and never provides answers to any real concern. I needed to focus on the discussion for the show, and Montel would take care of the rest. After all, it wasn't his first television show. Prior to the show, his staff called every day to check in and answer any questions. They seemed to understand my need for repetition of details, perhaps to ensure that I showed up in the right city and at the correct television studio.

As Terri and I waited backstage in our "Green Room," which is actually green, I continued to review my written talking points. As I glanced through the few pages of handwritten notes, I realized that my scanning was as vacant as the empty lunch basket sitting on the table next to me. Even though I had been living with cognitive disability, it wasn't always simple to quantify the experience in sound bites. There was a variety of chocolate spilling out of the basket, so I grabbed a handful of Hershey Kisses.

"My brain is full and closing," I said. "Maybe a sugar rush will help."

"Skip the notes," said Terri, "let's just talk through some of their sample questions." There was no way to know what Montel would ask us, so why worry about it, but I wanted to give direct answers about MS cognitive overload and not waste the opportunity. Working off my notes had added a difficult step to the discussion, so I put down the pages and never looked at them again. I found that my mind was trapped in analyzing the written question and unable to quickly move into a coherent response. Listening to a question was much easier and allowed me to step over a cognitive pitfall. Our private, green, guest room was comfortable and since we had several hours before the taping, we took turns bouncing interview questions off each other. Short and detailed answers would work for me, even if the chocolate ran out.

During the prior week, I had numerous telephone interviews by the show's staff, discussing details about the book and our choice of clothing for the show. I asked about the backstage temperature and the heat from the CBS Paramount studio lights, wondering how they would affect my MS-torched nerves. The cameras, live audience, and discussion with Montel didn't concern me, but being overheated by the dozens of spotlights gave me pause. Flaring up my MS symptoms on national television could mentally jam my thoughts, leaving me on the set with make-up and hair in place but unable to do much else other than point at the book. Ironically, being unable to place two sentences together would make a clear MS cognitive point.

"He keeps it absolutely freezing backstage and on the set!" said Stacey. She may not have understood Montel's reasoning for the arctic environment, but I felt an MS connection with him. As Terri and I were escorted through the studio's catacombs to sit down behind the set, I listened to the other guests squeal as they sat down and "discovered" the seemingly frozen grey metal chairs. I smiled. It was so pleasantly cold backstage that the other guests began to sniffle and wipe their noses with tissue. The make-up lady returned to touch up the streaks on each nose, covering lines that were marked from the tissue wipe. Show business is interesting.

While waiting backstage for my entrance cue, I could watch Montel on a monitor, warming up the audience and talking about the various efforts to calculate the true MS population. Whether the differing numbers belong to the National Multiple Sclerosis Society, the Centers for Disease Control and Prevention, or pharmaceutical companies, the number of people with MS is clearly growing. It is difficult to bring up the subject of MS in a conversation without learning about someone who was recently diagnosed with the disease. For people with newly diagnosed MS, we cannot undo the medical truth of their discovered lesions, but there is a long-term reality worth keeping in mind.

There is good news and bad news that accompanies the diagnosis of MS. The bad news is that it is a disabling and progressive disease without a cure. The good news is that people typically don't die from MS and may live as long as the non-MS population. Based upon what seems to be an undesired growing population, Montel strongly believes that the MS number is underestimated and possibly reaches one million in this country alone. Whatever the number may be, I agree with Montel that it is much higher than the government estimates and that its unabated growth is disturbing.

When Montel decided to introduce my book to his wide television audience, he was specifically sharing it with the majority of the MS population—whatever the number. When people with MS struggle to understand their cognitive challenges—why their memory recall and mental processing are being delayed and twisted—ascertaining an accurate number of affected individuals may be a vital, yet secondary, concern for them. Acknowledging MS cognitive impediments and disability, propelling the discussion into the mainstream of MS consciousness, Montel was leaping beyond the numbers debate. That public format validated MS cognitive struggles for people, opening a path for moving beyond the stealth symptoms to understanding and informed treatment.

While waiting for an entrance cue, I listened to Montel introduce me to the camera and 200+ member audience as they watched the video montage that was filmed at our Eastside home in Milwaukee. Montel was talking about how my legal career was shut down by cognitive symptoms of MS, but I couldn't absorb the details of what he was saying and ignored the moment. My ability to take in his comments about me was limited as I glanced at the quiet backstage movements of the production crew, hustling like an accelerated catering staff at a large wedding. Although the technical aspects of the show were fascinating to observe, I knew that everything must be tuned out. The cognitive limitations of my MS had taught me that, at best, I could only focus on one thing at a time. Shaking off this surreal moment, it would be a conversation with Montel.

"Are you ready for this?" asked Terri, as two stage-crew members prompted me to the few steps leading up to the set entrance.

"Just two guys with MS talking about the cognitive challenges," I answered. When the sliding doors opened onto the set, I was immediately met with Montel's smile and a gesture to sit in the chair next to him. As I crossed the set, I could sense the stares from the audience as they sat motionless and silent. Since the tan cloth furniture was familiar to me from watching the show on television, it felt like I had stepped into a comfortable memory that I had never previously experienced.

"Not fair!" I thought. Terri and I had been specifically told to not wear sweats or jeans on the show. As I shook hands with Montel and sat down, I noticed that he was wearing blue jeans. Of course, it was his television show, and we didn't want the interview to appear as if we were sitting on a park bench, but his casual style confirmed my decision to skip the socks.

"I'm really glad that you're here," said Montel. "Unfortunately, in this country, we look at illness as weakness, so if you can't see a physical manifestation of weakness, then you think that a person is not ill. With this disease, MS," Montel continued, "and with some of us, the physical manifestations aren't necessarily the first things that you come across." We dove right into a startling and invisible example of MS cognitive delay.

"It was just so profound when you talked about going into court one day," said Montel. The tense memory of my cognitive *loss of presence* during a court hearing felt fresh in my mind. "And sitting down at the table," continued Montel, "and the judge wanting you to start and you didn't even recognize your client as your client." I recounted how I struggled to understand my notes and why a client for two years suddenly appeared different and unfamiliar. As I described how I awkwardly pushed through the hearing to a successful conclusion, Montel smiled and pumped his fist as if saying "Yes—keep fighting!"

During the first commercial break, I began to scan the faces of the audience. Either out of respect or by instruction, they remained silent and bounced their stares at both me and Montel. While the lights went down a bit and the recording paused, the crew hustled to make technical adjustments. The gaze of the audience remained steady and gave me the sensation of being on the inside of a live museum exhibit. I caught the intense expressions of a young couple sitting together next to a woman in a wheelchair. Their concerned frowns were curious and supportive, as if saying "hang in there" and "don't stop." I smiled back at them and shrugged my shoulders in an effort to show that it wasn't a spinal tap procedure and that I appreciated their interest.

The commercial pause would have been a perfect opportunity for Montel to step off stage and take a break from the filming, but he stayed seated and never took his eyes off of me. Our real conversation was about to start. Montel remained seated with me and continued to ask about the book's cognitive discussion and how I was dealing with staving off further mental stumbles. Suddenly, his expression was intense and concerned while his voice became hushed and more directed between us. The cameras were still, and he spoke below the commotion level of the studio while audience members attempted to lean in to our quiet conversation.

Montel wanted to talk to me—without the camera recording. Although his message was not top secret, it was personal. He hunched forward a bit toward the edge of his chair, bringing our eye-to-eye contact even closer. The tumultuous sea of studio and audience activity continued to roll but became a quiet din against our conversation.

"I was wondering," asked Montel, "have you ever thought about learning to play piano?" He was excited about the suggestion and talked about the value of exercising the mind by pushing its current boundaries. As he shared his thoughts about encouraging the brain to find new ways to connect, Montel's eyes sparked with the anticipation of introducing a friend to a new delicious recipe with, "wait until you taste this!"

"Funny you ask," I answered, "but last week I was looking through our girls' piano lesson books and started tinkering with the introductory lessons. Lessons may be frustrating to me at this point, but I've always wanted to learn how to play." I reached out my right hand toward Montel and stretched my fingers to show the wide range between the far fingertips. As I tried to relax my hand and calm down the MS tremor, I visualized the nine to 10 keys that fit within the grasp. Learning to read music and translating the notes into keyboard movements would be a private exercise routine for my brain, rather than a rehearsal for a spring piano recital. Montel watched as I clasped my quivering hands back together and rested them back on my lap. He nodded his head and smiled as if saying, "I think you can do it."

Montel explained the importance of keeping his mind active and that the challenge to play piano is a great mental exercise. He wouldn't follow anyone's suggestions to take it easy and sit back, do nothing, and deteriorate. His philosophy was fashioned from pursuing strength, and Montel insisted that the mind must always be given something to work on, using both sides of the brain and connecting the thought process with some physical coordination—like playing the piano. Whether this meant linking a mental process to physical dexterity or another cognitively expressive outlet, it was mutually supporting a new bridge toward growing the neurologic routes of the brain.

As I shifted in my seat to face Montel, I noticed over my left shoulder that the studio's large flat-screen monitor hanging from the back of the set was displaying the cover of my book. Although optic neuritis had fogged my vision, the colors of the book were brilliant against the bronze-orange colors of the show's logo. Below the giant screen was a dark wood credenza with only one object resting on it. Tightly fit inside a framed triangle was a military-folded American flag. Given Montel's service background, I assumed that it was presented to him and serves as a proud statement of his training and commitment to this country.

When Montel attended the Naval Academy, he continued his bodybuilding training, side-by-side with pursing mental fitness. During his years of active military service, he studied both Chinese and Russian. Montel was commissioned as a cryptology officer and served on board both the *USS Kitty Hawk* and *USS Halsey*. No doubt the active challenge of intercepting, translating, and analyzing communications required a disciplined mind, and as Montel related in his book *Climbing Higher*, his work with the intelligence team on board would "provide data crucial to identifying two Libyan fighter aircraft that had crossed the 'line of death,' making an aggressive move toward one of our aircraft, and we shot them both down."

What may have been originally grounded in Montel's personal experience from analyzing multi-task communications in life-and-death moments, continues in his determination to take the fight to the enemy, in this case, a progressive disease. Whether he wanted to outreach his cognitive techniques from the personal experience of cognitive stonewalls or his reflections from reading my book, Montel understood what people with MS were cognitively enduring. He wanted to openly place his tactics in front of me and the MS community, an effort that seemed more important than not being able to wear jeans. The suggestions were a reflection of Montel's confidence and strength.

This was not part of an interview for a television show; it was personal. Montel knew something about successful MS cognitive strategies, and he wanted to exchange information. Before we arrived in New York, I wondered how Montel had managed any cognitive affects of MS. Most individuals with MS may not be significantly impaired by the cognitive symptoms, but they may struggle with interference in holding their thoughts in place. Montel had interviewed thousands of guests and managed a successful television career and family. Even without a disabling neurologic disease in tow, living in the spotlight as a television talk show host should tax anyone's brain connections to the extreme.

To whatever degree Montel may have dealt with cognitive delay and uncertainty, he would take action without hesitation, even if it meant exerting more mental effort. Through his mental-exercise regimen, he had found the means to think clearly in the eye of his own mental hurricane of demands. Perhaps, it was no different to him than a weight-lifting workout to increase muscle strength and endurance. Any maintenance of cognitive functions does not occur in a vacuum with wishful thinking. Sometimes it requires discovering new methods of mentally "exercising" very different places of the brain.

He had personal questions to ask about my MS cognitive experiences but also wanted to share, one person with MS to another. Although he could have been distracted by the numerous interruptions and activity by his staff, Montel never shifted his focus away from our conversation. Without losing eye contact between us, we had a conversation that was as comfortable as sitting and chatting in a coffee shop near my home. Just two guys sitting on nice living room furniture, talking about coping with MS, right?

"You could also try to study a foreign language," Montel continued. "It brings in areas of the brain not being used." He spoke about taking the mind to uncharted thinking territory, opening up previously untapped areas of the brain. "If encouraged, the brain can rewire itself," he continued, "finding new connections." The brain could learn to find new approaches to a task, if prompted.

In his book, Montel emphasized finding personal "tricks," such doing math skills and learning to categorize things as a means to strengthen the brain. He wrote, "If we have memory problems, there are mental exercises we can do to help stimulate the areas of the brain where memory occurs." Whether a person enjoys crossword puzzles or reading articles and making notes to capture the details, Montel's message was clear: "sharpen your memory" and find the "tricks" that help you to memorize and recall information.

From his experiences as a naval intelligence officer, Montel had learned many languages and was certainly familiar with the mental sharpening that occurs by translating detailed information. Perhaps similar to learning to play piano, studying a foreign language required constant practice with deep focus and fine tuning. These were skills that an MS-stalled and sometimes confounded brain should regularly pursue.

It is impossible to know where Montel would be now without having developed methods to sharpen his mental edge, but they certainly provided him with the tools to function with MS and not watch his life from the sidelines. Montel may have accomplished so much only by being compelled to push hard against what others may have set as his MS limits. Exercising both his mind and body is a deliberate choice to overcome obstacles. Without taking specific action to sharpen the edges of your own mental processing, where will the potential cognitive disconnections from MS leave your thoughts?

Although Montel was offering successful strategies for pursuing cognitive stimulating lessons, as a means of connecting brain functions through unused channels, he was not suggesting that all people with MS should become French-speaking concert pianists. Certainly any given new cognitive lesson may not work or be of interest for all people with MS. When exploring a new cognitive aptitude, a person may have a better chance of succeeding and sustaining the new skill if the individual had a prior interest in the technique. Being pushed to pick up an undesired expertise without some underlying talent or interest may doom the effort to fail.

Without some natural curiosity or drive, sometimes combined with patient and professional instruction, the cognitive load may be further overwhelmed, providing more frustration and highlighting a person's MS short circuits. Montel's point was for people with MS to find constructive ways to motivate their thoughts to either maintain or seek alternate routes in the brain. Without a significant challenge to continue learning, people with MS will miss a significant opportunity to impede further cognitive deterioration. The best way to hold on to your current mental speed and grasp may be by frequently using your brain, but consider adding Montel's suggested discipline to also teach yourself new actions and skills. Promoting mental idleness offers no real strategy or solace in surviving cognitive roadblocks.

"Before we start again," said Montel, "would you like something to drink?"

"A glass of syrah would be really nice," I answered. Montel laughed and then noted that they only had water available on the set.

During the breaks, Montel could have easily stayed on the content of the book, but Montel wanted to reach out beyond the show. He asked me if I was familiar with an attorney friend of his who had MS, someone who was apparently experiencing cognitive difficulties, similar to the discussion revealed in my book.

Montel was concerned that his friend was having some difficulty acknowledging and dealing with his cognitive impediments, and since I was an MS-retired attorney, perhaps his friend could relate to my cognitive barriers.

Montel asked about the difficult moments that I had encountered as an attorney. When I explained the delayed recall, the struggle to follow conversations and track lost details, it reminded him of the frustration being faced by his friend. Montel's face looked determined to do something, but he didn't want to force the subject on his good friend. Even when close friends or relatives are having difficulties coming to grips with their cognitive issues, it may be awkward to open the subject.

"Would you be able to send a copy of your book to him?" asked Montel. "I will get his e-mail and address for you." Montel was interested in placing the cognitive discussion into the hands of his friend, as the best approach to prompting the discussion. I agreed to contact his friend with the limitation of not forcing the subject. That made sense to Montel and he appreciated any information that I could directly share with his friend. It would be up to the friend to take the subject to another step. This was my first live peer-support discussion in New York, and I had forgotten that it was Montel listening and asking for assistance.

The studio lights came back up to full intensity and with the hush from the crew, I assumed that we were back to the show. This out-of-body experience wasn't lost on me as I sat in the middle of a television production whirlwind, listening to Montel Williams up close, offering to share his cognitive-conditioning exercises. They seem to be working for him, I thought to myself.

Montel reintroduced the cognitive topic and without missing a beat, the show snapped on and continued where we left off—wherever that was. It was becoming a struggle to not let the conversation slip into my mental fog that was now covering the audience, the floating cameras, and the line of production staff watching from the far walls.

Detecting an individual's cognitive obstructions may be impossible, since the delayed recall and mental stutters tend to be invisible to uniformed observers. A vacant head-nodding stare may hide a stunning mental jam and a *loss of presence*. Montel was certainly aware of my limitations, and he did not hesitate to back me up, even during the taping of the show.

"Are you still with me?" asked Montel, in a subdued voice under the audience applause. As he leaned in even further, while never losing eye contact, I nodded back to him. The days of preparation for the show and intense preproduction interviews may have taken a toll on my connectivity to the moment, but the pause allowed me to snap back for the next question. As a woman in the front row folded her arms for warmth, I knew that the combination of frigid air-conditioning and an endless chocolate fix had invisibly fueled our segment of the show.

"Now, you have been with us for this whole interview," asked Montel, "right?" Nodding my head, I felt fortunate that Montel didn't ask any questions outside of our backstage quizzing. It was good timing that Montel checked in on me, and it allowed my thoughts to unclog. The pace of the show, assisted by editing, flowed in a manner that waited for my thoughts to click in and kept me in the interview. Bracing for the inconsistency of cognitive shutdown, I was thankful for the supportive cadence of the interview with built-in commercial breaks to mentally breathe. Montel's sensitivity to my saturated mind was appreciated and the concern reflected his true soul.

When Montel announced to the studio audience that they were each receiving a copy of my book, it fulfilled my desire that this show's MS cognitive conversation would echo in the homes of people with MS and their families. The ripple effect of Montel's discussion would be meaningful and validating to the MS community.

Perhaps this was the core meaning of the title of his book, *Climbing Higher*. The words infer action and not stopping, especially with MS where the *mountain* may seem to grow as you climb. It is the sensation of being compelled to endlessly walk up the stairs of a down escalator. Even to attempt to maintain your current position with MS, you may need to keep moving up against the mountain. The only way to make progress is to pick up the "climbing" pace and, in the throes of cognitive challenges, add new angles to connect toward the summit. Cognitive exercises must be a constant fixture in maintaining a mental edge—to move higher.

As a volunteer peer supporter for the Wisconsin Chapter of the National Multiple Sclerosis Society, I have spoken with numerous people with MS about living successfully with this invasive disease. During the conversations, I can share what I have learned and suggest methods or materials for consideration that I and other people with MS have found useful and effective. A peer supporter does not have all of the answers, nor can one assume that any successful coping method may work for any other person. However, if I can place the tools for finding answers in people's hands, they may have a better opportunity to manage their MS.

There is an unspoken benefit received by many peer supporters. By the end of the call, I have typically received something in return from the caller, whether or not they realize it. As the callers share their concerns and frustration regarding MS treatments and exacerbations, overlapped with family and employment issues, I frequently learn as much from the callers as they may have learned from my imparted information. My discussion with Montel was unexpectedly the same, although in reverse order. What started as purely a sharing opportunity for MS cognitive information, quickly turned into a face-to-face peer support discussion and more.

Although I could only hope that the millions of viewers were able to better understand the cognitive aspects of MS and that the MS-related community would embrace the discussion, I did not anticipate that the embrace would be mutual. In fact, I walked away from the taping with an infusion of commitment and strength to push my cognitive awareness and exercise in different directions. It was about adopting new tactics.

When the taping finished, the audience was quickly escorted out of the studio, and the lights were lowered on the hustling staff and lingering guests.

"I really appreciate this opportunity to make the MS cognitive topic so public," I said to Montel.

"Thank you both for coming here," answered Montel, "and for writing a book about such a real part of MS. I think we handed out every available copy to the audience, a couple hundred." All I could do was exchange a hug with Montel. His solid arms and strong hands were like a grasp of compassion, quietly saying "be strong." Individuals like Montel, with his intense passion and sheer force of commitment to end MS, will help drive this disease out of people's lives and into mere history.

Two days later, I found myself at home sitting on the piano bench and glancing through *Piano Adventures-1A*. No one cared that I was wearing a t-shirt, jeans, and no socks.

Mental Sharpening Stones and Perspectives

1. Maintain your mental activity by challenging your mind with learning new skills. It may be the most effective way to keep your thoughts sharp and recall flowing.
2. Great mental exercise can take the form of studying a new language, which requires cognitive connections of translation through reading, pronunciation, and writing. These same skills are tapped in learning to play an instrument, such as the piano. Doing so with personally meaningful tunes may use the emotional regions of the brain, mentally coordinating with physical dexterity for the hands and feet.
3. Seek out diverse and cognitively stimulating lessons of interest to you.

4. Select a language or musical tune that touches your emotions and makes you smile.
5. Avoiding physical exhaustion may also prevent mental fatigue and loss of focus. For example, physically overheating your body may also leave your brain with a dragging, slow-to-absorb-information sensation.
6. Allow yourself mental breaks and take them whenever available.
7. Share your MS cognitive impediments and your successful strategies with those who may benefit from your experience. Explaining your learned techniques to others will allow you to not only realize the benefits to yourself, but accurately convey the strategies.

Sharpening with Grace

A Conversation with Mary Mullarkey

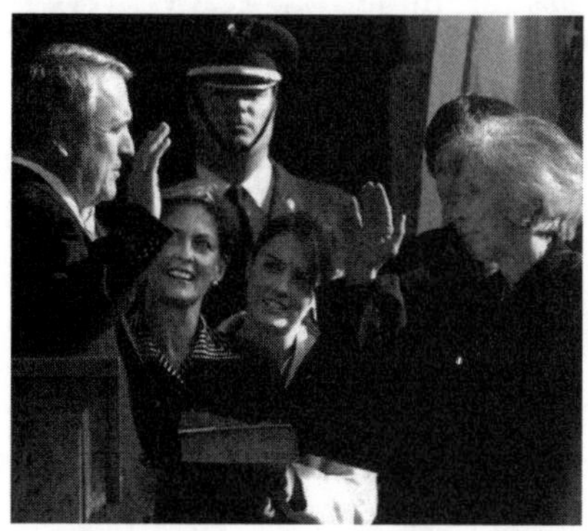

Mary Mullarkey is the Chief Justice of the Colorado Supreme Court. She shares how her use of cutting-edge computer technology, exercise, and a mentally challenging regimen has assisted her to maintain the speed and clarity required by her position—staying ahead of MS.

"One time I fell down before 300 people as I was making my way to the podium," said Mary Mullarkey, Chief Justice of the Colorado Supreme Court. Shaking off the tumble, she got up and reached the podium to present her speech. Although Mullarkey is faced with the challenges of MS, her perseverance is especially honest and laudable for managing MS while successfully integrating coping strategies into her personal and professional life.

Diagnosed with MS in 1994, Mullarkey was appointed to the Supreme Court of Colorado in 1987, where she learned to manage her MS symptoms and limitations, while leading the most powerful court in the state of Colorado. Mullarkey has no intention of allowing MS to slow her down or let it interfere with her judicial charge. Her style has never been to hide with fear from MS and, instead, she has sought out and readily accepted accommodations, which have allowed her to excel with grace. For Chief Justice Mullarkey, MS is a daily reality, but it has never been a reason to slow down on the court's bench or skip the details of life.

With the possible exception of the Rocky Mountains, the Colorado winters may remind Mullarkey of her childhood in Wisconsin. She grew up in New London, a town west of Green Bay, Wisconsin. It is an area known for both football and a frozen tundra named Lambeau Field. The wind-chill factor of Wisconsin winters reaches far below zero and is normally below the temperature in your freezer. It was in that seemingly arctic environment that Mullarkey learned to ice skate as a child.

"I used to go every night after school," said Mullarkey, "It was something you did." After shaking off a little rust from the passage of time, skating can be like riding a bicycle because you never really forget how to do it. It would be years later, while living in Colorado, that Mullarkey first realized that her skating wasn't the same. "We were out here in the mountains and I hadn't done it for a while, but I could not stand up on skates." Although many people may struggle on ice skates, this was different. Her balance was off and she kept going backward. It was this awkwardness and difficulty with balancing that tipped her off that there was something seriously wrong. The blades were not to blame.

She had faced unexplained physical symptoms, such as numbness in her feet and her arm, and had been steered toward misdiagnosis. The physical difficulties indicated a serious problem, but remained undiagnosed until 1994 when a neurologist informed her that she had MS. With an accurate diagnosis finally in hand, Mullarkey's unflappable determination to fulfill her judicial responsibilities was best evidenced by the action of the other justices of the Court, who in 1998, chose her to be the first woman Chief Justice of the Colorado Supreme Court.

In her role as Chief Justice, Mullarkey proudly represents the state's 275 judges and justices, supported by more than 2,800 full- and part-time employees of the Colorado Judicial Department. It is a position that Mullarkey embraces, demonstrating her strong leadership and practical insight, despite the MS that shadows her existence.

"We resolve every dispute that comes before us, no matter how difficult, no matter how emotional, no matter how volatile," she said during her 2007 speech on the *State of the Judiciary*. Whether listening to oral arguments along with her fellow justices, reviewing appellate briefs or drafting opinions, Mullarkey understands that each case presents its own legal world. The participants are due full consideration by the court, and there is no room for cutting corners or excuses offered for not properly managing the caseload or administration of the judicial system. Working in a system full of attorneys, the details are everything, and Mullarkey holds herself to the highest standards.

Holding Mental Balance

Approximately 1,400 new cases were filed in the Supreme Court during 2006, with disputes ranging from minor traffic infractions to multi-million dollar complex transactions, murder and drug cases, and seemingly everything in between. The volume of cases and the various depths of controversy presented to the court are enough to make anyone lose a bit of sleep at night, even without the reminders of carrying the chronic load of MS lesions. Instead of seeking relief from the mental demands of her position through moments of silent rest in her chambers or at home, Mullarkey has found balance for her MS symptoms through maintaining an exercise routine that includes swimming, water aerobics, and yoga. Physical action can also mean mental relaxation.

"Yoga can take a lot of different dimensions," said Mullarkey, noting how much she enjoys the breathing aspects of it. As she described the way that yoga has allowed her to mentally unwind from the intensity of a "normal" judicial day, I reflected on a few simple lessons that I have also learned from yoga. For those who have not participated in a yoga class, there may be a misunderstanding about why anyone alive would need to "learn" how to breathe, especially when the method seems to come naturally. However, although most people tend to start life with an untaught breathing process, there is more to be learned from the technique beyond unconsciously forcing air in and out of the lungs.

Through local yoga classes in my neighborhood, I have also found an appreciation of the slow and deep flow of air into my body, best received by a welcoming seated posture and relaxed cognitive focus. Easing my thoughts, while only thinking through the drift of air flowing through my body, removes a lot of toxic mental clutter and sharpens my mind to deal with the real subjects than remain. Simply stated, yoga also stretches the mind.

Unlike many workout routines that may require specific equipment, expensive clothing or an exercise facility, I have found that the breathing aspects of yoga can be practiced in most places, whether in public or private spaces. Although the seated position can vary with each individual, as much as the style of the pillow that a person is sitting upon, untangling the mind is a common effect. Yoga may also increase physical flexibility and strength, but its ability to open mental avenues and release the sharpness of thoughts should not be ignored, regardless of the environment. For me, the breathing exercises can be practiced sitting on living room carpet or while endlessly waiting for an elevator. It is a portable cognitive skill, simple to connect with my body and regroup my thoughts. "Yoga is something that I do at home or in classes," said Mullarkey. "The yoga breathing is helpful, particularly relaxation techniques, and those can be done anywhere." Perhaps remember: there is always time to learn how to breathe.

Mullarkey appreciates that there is more than one benefit received from practicing yoga, acknowledging that it can invigorate the body while clearing and calming the mind. For many people who strive for the benefits of exercise, a "workout" can still be perceived as an increasing chore, an ever-exhausting distraction from the daily list of necessary burdens. It is certainly no different for those also dealing with the added impediments from MS. Seeking a different exercise pathway to obtain the benefits that she had previously received from walking, Mullarkey found that water aerobics and yoga have amply filled the void. Knowing this end result from her adapted exercise routine is motivation for Mullarkey to maintain the push to remain physically active.

"Lots of times I have to make myself do something, like go to water aerobics," said Mullarkey. "Then, after, I feel so much better." Her determination is focused on the positive long-range benefits of the water aerobics and yoga. "It's not always an absolute joy to do this stuff, but in the longer term, I think it really has good effects." Speaking specifically about the cognitive benefits, Mullarkey noted that a good workout increases her mental relaxation, "because you're concentrating on something totally different."

Mullarkey doesn't need to convince herself to exercise, even when there are days that she might rather sit still. However, the thought of skipping an exercise opportunity is fleeting, since she appreciates the greater sense of well-being that can come from pursuing different physical activities.

"If I do this," Mullarkey said, "I will feel better and I will enjoy it." With activities such as water aerobics and yoga, she has found a workout that holds her interest. Mullarkey emphasizes that people should create and seek various kinds of physical recreation activities that make it fun and interesting for themselves. The dual benefit from physical activity for both the mind and body does not occur in a vacuum of idleness. Without interest, they will be casually excused and eventually lost if the activities become too routine and boring.

She has found that physical exercise works hand in hand with exercising the brain. Mullarkey has always loved walking, and when she was unable to do that anymore due to MS, she understood that it was crucial to maintain both her mind and body through a sustained exercise routine. When she was faced with a limitation imposed by MS, it would have been too easy to do nothing about the loss of a physical ability. However, Mullarkey recognized that if she had accepted inactivity, it would equal two distinct losses: achieving physical capabilities and pursuing a mental calm. Instead, her body is better conditioned to push back against any encroaching MS impediments and her mind is relaxed to sharply focus on her judicial duties.

Although I am not a master of yoga or even capable of relaying even the most subtle techniques to others, I too have personally experienced the mental benefits noted by Chief Justice Mullarkey. What yoga position or breathing technique works best for either of us may be far different than what works for you, but the opportunity to ease your mind and stretch the pathways of your brain should be explored. Learning and practicing yoga can clear and link the pathways of the brain.

Exercising your mind can take many different modes. Mullarkey also enjoys attending shows at the repertory theatre, since this activity allows her to step back from the cognitive demands of her professional life, away from reviewing the stack of appellate briefs, absorbing oral arguments, writing decisions and administering the court system.

"Going to those [shows] takes me into some other forms of thinking," said Mullarkey, acknowledging that there is more than one method to stimulate the functions of the brain and that subscribing to a local repertory company can provide a variety of productions to invigorate the connections in any person's brain. For Mullarkey, it is an exceptional diversion from the expectations and atmosphere of her judicial position.

Similar to performing physical exercise, seeking mentally stimulating entertainment requires cognitive attention and effort. People should define for themselves the sort of productions that encourage and sometimes provoke the brain to continue contemplating the event, carrying the performance message into post-show conversation with friends. Prompting your brain to verbalize the experience with others—whether it is a Shakespeare or Marx Brothers production—allows your brain to reap the benefits of stimulating entertainment.

"This is not a nine-to-five kind of job," said Mullarkey, "and one of the things about it is the reading and writing and research job." Given the paperwork load for each appellate case, Mullarkey has to take a lot of material home to read. In addition to the oral arguments, each case may also have a number of exhibits, transcripts, correspondence and stacks of case history to review. Unfortunately, much of her enjoyment from reading other books and newspapers has been lost because of the intensity of legal scrutiny. "I don't do as much reading for fun as I would like to," said Mullarkey. "One of the things that this job ruins for you is that it's hard to turn off my proofreading monitor, reading word for word, checking for mistakes. That's one of the bad things about it."

While reading for pleasure may be quashed by the sheer mass of a chief justice's paperwork, focused on a detailed and considered review of thousands of written submissions, she finds no reason to write off other mental challenges. After all, the judicial surroundings are not the boundaries for her mind, nor do they utilize her full thought potential. Although conversations with friends can provide Mullarkey with engaging moments of mental interaction, she has also discovered that her passion for playing the piano has encouraged the use of other dimensions of the brain.

"That uses a whole different part of your brain, as far as I can tell," noted Mullarkey, "especially trying to memorize songs; that's really demanding when trying to figure out how the key movements work." Perhaps similar to the effortless-appearing movements of an Olympic gymnast, playing the piano often seems much easier than the true reality of the effort. The good players make it look simple, giving it a sense of an unconscious effort. "With the piano, there's a lot of thought about it," Mullarkey reflected. As far as the whole left side and right side of the brain are concerned, she has noted that the creative side of the brain that enables her to play the piano is different than the other side, which allows her to process legal issues.

Mullarkey strongly believes that playing the piano stimulates different pathways in the brain. Her theory makes sense, especially when considering the combination of reading the music, cognitively processing the visual notes, and translating them into a flurry of hand and finger movements. Mullarkey learned to play piano when she was a child, but the lessons have extended far beyond any written bars and chords printed on sheet music.

"It certainly teaches me something about dexterity," said Mullarkey. "I have enjoyed it and got even more into it the last few years." Mullarkey appreciates that her continued practice of piano has provided more than just music in her home, along with challenges to her hand and finger coordination. "It's the whole thing about how the brain works and which side is supposed to be the creative side," she continued, "and using each side seems to help the other side function." Recognizing and maximizing the number of connections in your brain may be a means to maintain cognitive function, learning even more when you enjoy the activity.

Sharpening Skills

Many individuals who play a musical instrument cannot overstate the significance of how playing the music lifts them into another level of mental connections. When I was a child, I enjoyed watching *The Andy Griffith Show* and was fascinated to see how the entire telephone system for the fictional town of Mayberry flowed through one switchboard operated by "Sarah." In the one-sheriff town, every call had to be manually connected by a black cable pulled from the receiving call board and plugged into the intended home or business socket, located on the board facing the operator. Through experience, Sarah knew whose telephone was represented by each open hole in the switchboard, and the connections were seemingly instant to the townsfolk, operating like a single brain.

When MS disrupts the "thinking" nerve connections in my brain, I have struggled to connect with the stored pieces of information located—somewhere. Whether trying to remember why I had walked into the kitchen or finding myself stuck in a word vacuum and unable to recall what I was saying, I have pictured Sarah in my brain, taking the cable from the requesting peg and trying to find the correct slot on a blocked and moving information board. If MS were a character on the show, it would be portrayed by a nasty kid who sneaks in behind Sarah and randomly pulls out the cables, severing communication connections in the town, allowing them to fall in a tangled pile on the floor. Every day, that MS kid would pull the same stunt, rendering the connections for even the simple thinking tasks randomly unreliable.

When MS lesions yank out the cables from my cognitive switchboard, I cannot force a quick rewiring. It often seems that the more I struggle to recall the lost words or recognize a location or face, the more difficult it becomes to grasp the knowledge that I had taken for granted. By routinely exercising my brain to find new "cables," whether by learning to play music or practicing yoga, I envision "Sarah" learning to use new cables, finding a new route to connect the call. Maintaining the connections and recognizing the options for adding new ones is an ongoing action for sharpening the brain.

Although it is a keen cognitive-sharpening skill, Mullarkey's interest in playing piano has provided more enduring meaning to her than simply mastering musical scales. "It's a form of expression, and you get a lot of satisfaction and emotion about playing piano," she noted. What started as a childhood experience has developed into an insightful understanding of the brain's ability to develop varied dimensions. She has embraced "the idea about using the other pathways of the brain," which sustain cognitive strength to fulfill her judicial activities. Not only is playing the piano an enjoyable skill to maintain for a lifetime, it is purposeful mental exercise, providing a connection for cognitive cables.

The life of a Supreme Court chief justice may be completely mentally draining by the end of each day. However, cognitive cross-training may be an effective method to strengthen the mind. Often you may observe that athletes who are highly skilled at one sport will cross-train their body and excel at a seemingly different physical activity. In their off-season, for example, speedskaters may become avid bicyclists. It is not merely because the outdoor scenery is more diverse than endlessly racing counterclockwise on an indoor 400-meter oval, but because the muscle and cardiovascular workout of bicycling compliments the skater's sprinting and distance speedskating.

Bringing underused physical attributes on line for the body may not only allow physical connections to operate more efficiently, but may also encourage the body to recognize and use otherwise ignored muscles. Exploring the full potential of the body's untapped tools to achieve physical goals is like modifying your driving style and obtaining better gas mileage with the same car.

The same concept of cross-training may be applied to cognitive exercises. With her lifetime love of playing piano and her practice of yoga breathing and relaxation, Mullarkey not only has challenged herself to maintain her current level of cognitive functions, but has welcomed new technology as a method of staying cognitively sharp and productive. From inside the Colorado Supreme Court, there may be no hint of a shrinking caseload; on the contrary, the judicial system may be bracing for an increase of filings and appeals.

Through her proactive efforts to seek new methods of effectively drafting her work, Mullarkey has been able to maintain her current work levels and do her work more efficiently with increased focus on the content of her writing. Throughout facing all of the personal changes that MS has compelled her to absorb, Mullarkey understands that dealing with the impediments doesn't have to be a one-person effort. The need for an accommodation may not always be evident, even to those who work closely with her, but remaining silent offers little opportunity for maintaining a current level of functioning, especially when the work is thrust into the public eye.

Welcoming Accessibility

When she was asked to officiate for swearing in the newly elected governor of Colorado, Bill Ritter, Mullarkey immediately began to contemplate her accessibility with a walker. "The ceremony always takes place on the landing of the west steps of the Capitol in January," recalled Mullarkey, "and the speakers' podium is built out and up a few precarious steps from the landing." She immediately realized that she would have to walk down 20 to 30 steps to her seat on the platform. "I was aware of the difficulties with the platform for the inaugural ceremony because I have attended many of the inaugural ceremonies and presided at two of them."

She immediately understood that advance notification and planning would be the key for a seamless formal ceremony. Accommodation doesn't always knock first, and without foresight, an MS moment can pose more than a little difficulty or embarrassment. Mullarkey took the initiative to investigate her accessibility for the ceremony and determine what obstacles existed and how they could be minimized or removed. "Given that the speakers' platform is built especially for the ceremony, I knew they could accommodate my concerns if I raised them early enough."

Two weeks before the inauguration, she spoke with her staff about adjusting the stage to ease her approach with a walker. "People are very willing to help," noted Mullarkey, "but if you don't think of it until the last minute, it can make it very hard for them to undo things." In this case, there were no steps to reach the speakers' podium, and the accommodation was having a ramp. This access could not have been modified with short notice.

The swearing-in ceremony for the governor is traditionally held outside in January, regardless of the Colorado weather. Logistically, it can be quite challenging for Chief Justice Mullarkey to get from one building to another because of all of the snow. "Our building is kitty-corner, across the street from the Capitol," she noted. "To get from here to there was quite a challenge because of all of the snow." When she spoke with the security guards well in advance of the ceremony, they understood her situation and told her that they would make sure to assist her mobility, including escorting her onto the stage. Mullarkey had no concern about being at the correct location at the right moment when the governor raised his hand.

Accommodation can take time and planning, both requiring advance notice of the need. Curves on a mountainous road are better dealt with when there is advance signage for forthcoming sharp turns. Once you have missed the turn, it may be too late to avoid plunging off the cliff. For someone who needs a bit of accommodation, it's far better to say something up front, rather than wait until it's too late, causing twice the effort because now others have to undo something before proceeding with the task at hand.

However, a strategic tool for accommodation is rarely plopped onto anyone's desk without the person first expressing a need and willingness to welcome a new method of practice. In fact, one of Mullarkey's best coping strategies for her work at the Supreme Court was found by asking for a bit of help, making a change that would allow her to maintain her responsibilities. By doing so, Mullarkey has exemplified the concept that acknowledging a need for assistance and seeking a practical accommodation is a powerful tool to cope with obstacles.

Although the simplicity of seeking available tools to accomplish your goals may seem obvious to some, many people could use a reminder about the personal benefit received by asking for and accepting the assistance. "Going it alone," rather than finding and accepting a new strategy for ongoing success, tends to draw more attention to the struggle. As Chief Justice of the Colorado Supreme Court, Mullarkey has no intention of letting MS play an interfering role.

Learning a New Language

One of the most significant changes that Mullarkey made at her work was intended to ensure that the vital timing of her opinion drafting, as well as intrajudicial and administrative correspondence, would never by compromised due to MS hurdles. She had learned about verbal "hands-free" software programs and researched the options for integrating the system with the computer in her chambers. The software would allow her to dictate faster than she could type, especially because she is limited by MS numbness in her hand, slowing her dexterity. As fast as she could clearly state the words into the computer's microphone, the software would recognize each word and process it into a corresponding word to be viewed on the screen.

Integrating technologic change can take time and patience, but the benefit is worth the temporary aggravation of mastering the technology. Once Mullarkey obtained technical assistance to load the program on her computer, the burden shifted to her to learn how to use the interactive system. This was no small task and was an extra personal commitment, since the computer must also learn to understand the individual's spoken words. No one compelled Mullarkey to discover or accept the use of this advanced program, and the responsibility for establishing the communication with the computer belonged to her alone. Mullarkey understood that this was a well-spent investment of her time.

For the user and computer, the interpreted dictation is a learned task, as a parent might teach a child to understand words and tone. When the user and computer are in sync, the program will "listen" and automatically translate an individual's spoken words immediately into typed text, without loss of the speaker's thought context. What had been thought of as a bit of science fiction from an old episode of the television show *Star Trek*, is now common reality and widely available to the consumer.

"It's a pretty sophisticated program," said Mullarkey, noting that the English versions include American, British and Indian. Although the words may be the same, the accents can be interpreted differently by the program. "You've got to talk to it and read text," Mullarkey continued, "and then it corrects and updates your vocabulary and your personal accent. It did take time to train the software to identify my voice and speaking patterns," said Mullarkey, but this process allows the program to work more precisely. The program is also self-monitoring and updates itself whenever she uses it. Whether Mullarkey uses the program to dictate e-mails or letters or to draft legal opinions, it saves her valuable time and increases the accuracy of capturing her thoughts and placing them into print.

"The voice-activated software is really wonderful," she continued. "It's so fast!" Her voice held the enthusiastic excitement of a person who discovers that her car's gas mileage has far exceeded the car dealer's representations. Realizing that this hands-free program has allowed her to bypass an MS limitation and "type" documents at an accelerated speed—perhaps faster than her own best typing—Mullarkey has no intention of going back to the old typing method. By learning the verbal program at this point in her judicial career, Mullarkey has successfully taken preemptive action to avoid a possible future interference due to MS.

This reminds me of a dear artistic friend, Sally Fogelberg, who intentionally taught herself to work ambidextrously. Whether completing her award-winning pen-and-ink drawings or acclaimed quilting, she could work with either hand leading the way. Sally didn't know what the future might bring, but she wasn't going to let her gifted abilities vanish if her hand was injured. When she had a stroke in 2007, incapacitating one side of her body and rendering one hand still, the other side was prepared to continue her artistic efforts. Since Sally had trained both sides of her brain and body to interpret and accomplish the same task, her artistry may be impeded but not silenced. Through years of self-training her brain to cross-over her skills to the "other" side of the brain, she caused it to find other neurologic paths to perform the same function. It was the same purpose through different routing. This would have been a daunting task to accomplish during her post-stroke recovery, but she invested the energy and time, connecting those cognitive cables, well in advance of the need.

Although few people can anticipate the timing and consequences of a traumatic health event to their body, it is not impossible to take advance precautions to protect the abilities that are most valued—whether cognitive or physical. When the mind or body seems to be functioning at its best is perhaps the ideal time to learn alternative methods of performing the same task or to find the means to improve the efficiency of the accomplishment. This strategy is a means to be prepared for that additional and sometimes unanticipated cognitive demand.

Mullarkey faces down the demands of her legal work by pacing out the workload and not trying to pin the effort to a "normal" workday. She has two law clerks and a clerical assistant to help her stay on top of the active caseload. Although she works with her clerks on the legal opinions, the verbal software program allows her to draft documents by herself and without clerical help. Even with the assistance of her staff, Mullarkey's "typical" day is anything but typical. The aggregate commitment to work through the volume of each case file results in Mullarkey pushing her hours beyond a 9-to-5 day. Her desk often substitutes as a lunch table, with the food bordered by case files.

During the same day, she may also read pleadings and briefs, combined with reaching decisions and voting on five different cases. In between, she may participate in several short meetings and phone conversations, dealing with ongoing administrative matters. This may include hiring a key employee and authorizing adequate money for the attorney-client protection fund (which reimburses clients whose monies have been stolen by attorneys), as well as approving the plans for a new state judicial building. She may be simultaneously working with one law clerk to finalize a dissent to another justice's opinion, while working with her other law clerk on the draft for a different opinion, that she is writing. In between all of this activity, she may meet with one of her colleagues to discuss a case that he is working on and in the remaining moments, check her e-mail. Any extra time gained through use of the verbal software is obviously valuable to Mullarkey.

For Mullarkey, managing her judicial time is not only a necessity for timely processing the case load and administering the court, but also a means to avoid placing extra stress on her MS symptoms. Saving time is a potent strategy that can be best achieved when it is hooked up with technology that affords a more efficient use of cognitive skills. Of course, once a technology is integrated into a person's routine, maintaining or excelling the person's abilities, there is a sort of welcomed dependence that may occur and may have to be acknowledged.

If the verbal software program suddenly malfunctioned and weren't available, the system's failure wouldn't bring Mullarkey's work to a halt. Although the use of verbal software is now part of her method of written communication, Mullarkey understands that she would find some other way of coping. "I can certainly do short memos, but any kind of longer documents—I don't know." If compelled to do so, she would probably go back to simple handwriting and although much slower, and would accurately record her thoughts; there are, however, definite speed limits to handwriting, as compared with using the software. More than likely, she would need to use a secretary, which would also slow down the accustomed speed of her work. Fortunately, it doesn't appear that the software will be obsolete any time soon.

When I suggested that communicating with the program is a good partnership, almost like being married, Mullarkey agreed, with the exception that "it can't quite finish my sentences." The program also allows the user to still type with the keyboard, which enables Mullarkey to use the keyboard for commands and corrections. Although it took some time for the program to become familiar with Mullarkey's voice, the benefits of increased speed of typing far outweigh any time invested in changing her established drafting methods. By accepting the new technology, she has gained far more than she has lost.

"It types so much faster," said Mullarkey. "This is almost instantaneous, and that's a big improvement." For most people who type, "almost instantaneous" is an unimaginable speed improvement over finger-pecking at a keyboard. The fact that the program also spells the dictation correctly is an enhancement over the typical style of "close-enough" typing, until you run the spellchecker. Of course, most people have learned that a spellchecker cannot catch the wrong word, if it is typed correctly as a different word—"if" when you meant to type "of." None of this would occur with verbal software.

Mullarkey is the first justice on the Colorado Supreme Court to use a voice command program, and she doesn't hesitate to suggest that others may realize the benefits from accepting its assistance. She encourages other people with MS to explore whatever technical options might be available to assist them in facing high cognitive-stress demands. Learning a new technology may itself be quite challenging, but once mastered, the technology can preserve or enhance a skill level.

"I have often found that the technological things that make life easier turn out to be so much work to learn," said Mullarkey. However, she was pleasantly surprised by the end result and, in this case, the increased speed justified the added time and aggravation of teaching a computer to recognize her verbal commands. "Its regression and progression," she said. And, in the case of the Chief Justice of the Colorado Supreme Court, one step backward to learn new technology was worth countless steps forward.

When asked about the reaction she received as the first justice to request the additional software and training, Mullarkey said that there was no hesitation by the court's technical support staff to step in and get the program up and effectively running for her. "People are more than willing to try to help, but do not offer because they don't want to be intrusive," said Mullarkey. "People may think that it's work to speak up to ask for assistance." However, mind reading is not a learned skill, even for those with a true desire to assist. Whether accessibility means providing a ramp or software, asking for help with the connection is acceptable and encouraged.

Connecting the Gap

Often, people with MS who are dealing with cognitive moments of stalled or confounded thinking may find that it is too complicated to describe the difficulty to others and simply prefer to punch their way through the mental cobwebs, sometimes being tangled into the mental muck. Some who may wish to ask for assistance with their moments of cognitive disconnection don't know how to ask for help or where to turn for assistance for specific strategies. Clear memories may temporarily be difficult to grasp on demand and seem invisibly blocked from articulation. To recover from the disappearing act that my thoughts may take, I have found another technologic trick to preserve what is on the tip of my tongue.

Similar to Chief Justice Mullarkey's use of verbal software as a means to quickly and accurately record her dictated work, a free and easily accessible method is available for everyone to hold onto their thoughts. If not quickly recorded in some manner, the thought may be lost. Whether the thought was vital, precious, or trivial, forgetting what I was thinking or being unable to recall a detail is a daily side-effect of my cognitive interference from MS. It is like placing a thought into a bottle and then setting it floating into a fast-flowing river and looking away for just a moment. When I turn back to look at the same location on the river, the bottle is long gone, somewhere. Of course, people with MS cannot walk around connected to verbal software, recording their meaningful dictation on instant notice.

Or can they?

As a useful cognitive strategy, many individuals will call home or their own cell phone and leave a voicemail message for themselves with either a good hint or a detailed discussion to be recalled when they later check for messages. That can be very effective, unless someone at home is using the phone and the voicemail is inaccessible or "full" for whatever reason. In those situations, delay upon delay only adds to the derailing of the train of thought. The next step of improvement is to transfer your thoughts directly to your computer, although you are nowhere near the keyboard.

The availability of verbal software to be used on the run is more within reach than many realize. For those who may cognitively struggle to hold their thoughts until paper and pen are available or are impatient waiting for a computer to boot up, using *Jott.com* is a practical strategy to preserve those bits of information that may not survive until a recording device is at hand.

By spending a few moments on line at the Jott.com site, you can register your phone or phones so that the site's phone number recognizes that you are calling. It will allow you to speak in 30-second units, while its built-in verbal software automatically types your stated words and forwards them in a message to your e-mail address or text message (if you speak that "language"). When you need to leave multiple messages, the technology is flexible. It is verbal-recognition software that travels with you.

There is no way to guarantee that Jott.com will indefinitely exist in its current structure, but it is a valuable tool and evidences a technologic trend that should be available in some manner, if you search for it and make it work for you. Asking for assistance can be the means to continue functioning in a similar manner and also beyond past expectations.

When Chief Justice Mullarkey presented the *State of the Judiciary* speech to the Colorado legislature in January of 2007, she used a walker when the legislators ceremonially escorted her in the House of Representatives. She had dictated her speech using the verbal software that she had become accustomed to using in writing her legal opinions. Through seeking and welcoming assistance for her physical challenges, Mullarkey has refused to forego the rich opportunities of her career and life. Through sharpening her mind with the influence of playing piano and yoga, while also enjoying thought-engaging social activities, Mullarkey has calmly sharpened the edges of her mind, outside of the demands of her judicial venue. Her use of verbal software has ensured that the speed and accuracy of her drafting will not lose a step.

"We convince ourselves that we have nothing to lose," said Mullarkey, "by staying at home and pulling the covers over our heads." However, she has demonstrated that without taking risks, even when faced with potential mistakes, we would miss out on the greatest accomplishments of our lives. Embracing technologic strategies such as learning to master verbal software, Mullarkey has not merely endured living with MS, but has thrived by leading with judicial grace and serves as an exemplar of staying ahead of the MS cognitive roadblocks. She urges individuals to not be held back and instead, to be hopeful and "fill your lives with courage and determination." Her pursuit of judicial and personal goals through exercising her mind and improving its efficiency is a persuasive method to stay out of the shadows of MS impediments.

Chief Justice Mullarkey's position has the compelling vigor of a legal opinion with no dissent.

Mental Sharpening Stones and Perspectives

1. Explore different mental exercises for each side of the brain to stimulate the connections. Physical and mental exercises can mutually support and benefit each another.
2. Identify an exercise routine or physical activity that provides stimulating movement for the body and stretches the mind to calmly focus on the flow of action. Concentrating on your physical exercise, whether aerobic or yoga, may provide different levels of mental relaxation.
3. Be determined to reach the long-term benefits of physical and mental exercise by varying the routine and avoiding the dullness of repetition.
4. Learn to read music and play a musical instrument. This may stimulate less-used mental pathways, recognizing and connecting "both sides" of the brain.
5. Explore new technology as a means to maximize your cognitive functions. Be sure to seek technical help to assist you in learning to use the software or devices.
6. Request mental or physical accommodations where useful, and provide as much advance notice as possible to those involved. Assistance is best provided with a timely request.
7. Seek and learn alternative methods for the same tasks if it allows you to function more efficiently and with less mental stress. By doing so, you may preserve or exceed a measured level of activity.

CHAPTER 2

A Neurologist's Thoughts on Thinking in Multiple Sclerosis

Eric Maas, MD

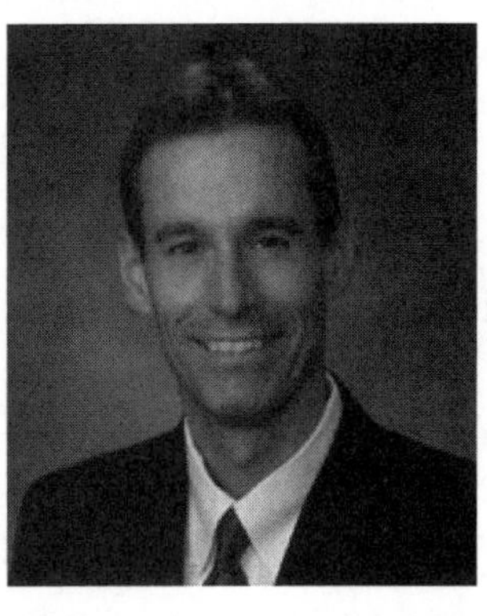

Dr. Maas is a neurologist in Milwaukee, Wisconsin, and is a member of the Clinical Advisory Committee of the Wisconsin chapter of the National Multiple Sclerosis Society. His clinical practice maintains a special interest in multiple sclerosis.

"Doctor, what do you mean 'silent' areas of the brain?"

A person recently diagnosed with multiple sclerosis (MS) often asks this question while reviewing magnetic resonance imaging (MRI) studies or while discussing the nature of inflammatory lesions affecting the white matter of the brain. This discussion should lead to the first mention of the cognitive deficits that may be caused by accumulated lesions in the brain's white matter.

In fact, there are numerous clinical scenarios in which the possible cognitive impairment due to MS should naturally be introduced as an aspect of the person's illness. I will illustrate a few of these clinical situations and patterns of recognizing and approaching MS cognitive problems. All neurologists and clinicians involved in the care of people afflicted with MS certainly have similar and additional experiences that they could share as well. However, the most important message to convey is that cognitive function in MS should be part of the ongoing discussion between people with MS and their physicians and should be a standard element of the person's continued evaluation and disease management.

Caring for patients with MS requires maintaining attention to the numerous aspects of how the illness affects individuals and dealing with the spectrum of diagnostic and management decisions. Keeping abreast of new scientific and clinical breakthroughs and bringing these new ideas and treatments safely to the care of appropriate individuals is essential in a neurologist's practice. During the last couple of decades, the cognitive deficits caused by MS have been more properly recognized and characterized. Despite early descriptions of altered mentation (the act of thinking) in MS patients dating back to Dr. Charcot in the mid 1800s, this key element of neurologic function threatened by the illness went relatively ignored for decades.

The cognitive deficits were thought to be a matter only for those patients most severely affected by other more-obvious physical deficits. During those many years, the changes in cognition (thinking skills such as perception, memory, awareness, reasoning, judgment, intellect, and imagination) seemed only to be recognized in patients with more severe and obvious cognitive impairment (a decrease in the ability to process, learn, and remember information). The deficits were only vaguely characterized as problems in memory and a feebleness of mind, along with an inappropriate jocularity or cheerful indifference to their situation and illness. However, most treating neurologists, patients, caregivers, and family members often recognized more subtle and important changes in cognitive function not restricted to these extremes.

Through the dedicated and insightful efforts of a few neuropsychologists who recognized this problem and had a particular interest in the manner in which MS might affect cognition, the character of these cognitive alterations, including the more subtle yet important deficits, began to be defined. The benefits of this work now provide a practical framework and clinical understanding that allows us to bring the evaluation of cognition into the proper place in the standard of care for those affected by MS.

Although the onset and course of many neurologic impairments in MS can be easily recognized, the cognitive deficits are usually more subtle in their onset and progression and, therefore, may elude detection for some time. Patients are often hesitant to mention cognitive concerns, and it is easy for physicians to overlook subtle deficits or to attribute them to fatigue or medication side-effects. This again underscores the importance of routinely including the direct discussion of cognitive performance as part of ongoing assessment.

Scenario One

Returning to the clinical scenario that I mentioned in the opening paragraph, this scenario illustrates what is probably the most common situation. Typically, physical or somatic symptoms have brought an individual to the care of a physician and then to the neurologist, where ultimately a diagnosis of MS is determined. Take for instance the presentation of an intensive care unit nurse with a young family who has a history of optic neuritis occurring a few years prior and now develops numbness over one half of her face and body. An MRI shows new inflammatory changes in the brain white matter in comparison to the MRI done at the time of her optic neuritis. Because no other abnormalities were found in her physical examination and blood tests, she is told that her symptoms fulfill the diagnostic criteria for MS.

In the course of the initial interactions with her neurologist, it would be unlikely that mention of any cognitive concerns would have immediately arisen. Then, as the discussions unfold regarding the rationale for treatment with immunomodulator medications and the need to have future MRI scans and visits for ongoing evaluation, the topic of cognitive function seems most naturally to become a point of review.

The appropriate time to raise the possibility that MS could affect mentation is part of the art of medical care. People have a myriad of questions and concerns when newly diagnosed with MS, and time needs to be taken to address each important issue. In the scenario above, if no cognitive concerns are raised by the patient or are apparent to the neurologist, then this discussion tends to come at a later visit.

But it needs to happen.

It should occur when a patient is ready to digest the information. This appropriate time varies from individual to individual and should arise early in their care. For example, it would be a timely discussion after people have had time to come to terms with the diagnosis, have accepted a treatment plan, and are ready to discuss the possible cognitive aspects of their illness.

When explaining the benefits of immunomodulator treatment in limiting white matter lesions and reducing the chances of brain atrophy, most patients readily move toward the subject of cognitive function. This often follows an explanation of the benefit in doing routine brain MRI scans in monitoring for new lesions that might have occurred, despite the absence of any new physical symptoms. These "clinically silent attacks" in the white matter may accumulate over time and contribute to cognitive impairment, as these areas of brain are not truly functionally silent. Rather, these areas involve pathways important in the transfer of information between various cortical regions of the brain. As you may imagine, it is natural that a discussion of possible cognitive injury due to MS would follow this explanation.

For the nurse described above, a self-assessment of how she has been doing in keeping track of the kids' schedules and household finances, her performance in stressful times on the job, and her continuing nursing education could be elements of a typical and appropriate initial discussion. This also allows for more comfort in raising the discussion again in the future and to help sort out normal experiences in lapses in memory and organization apart from that which may be more of a concern as being due to MS. Frequently patients will also then ask, "What could possibly be done if a deficit in the cognitive realm was truly suspected?" This opens the door to an explanation of the value in expert neuropsychological consultation and the fact that potential change in cognitive function should be as important as any other element of neurologic function threatened by MS in making decisions regarding medical treatment.

Scenario Two

Another scenario involves the patient who presents with mild to moderate recognizable cognitive disruption due to MS. It may be that a change in performance at work or home has lead to the first or subsequent neurologic evaluation. An elementary-school teacher who was previously diagnosed with MS had no residual symptoms or concerns and had not seen a neurologist for a number of years. She then decided to return for neurologic care when she thought that fatigue from MS might be affecting her life.

In reviewing her history, it was apparent that fatigue was an element of her problem but that other difficulties in multitasking, word finding, concentration, planning, and attention seemed to be more disordered than could be explained by the fatigue alone. Neuropsychological testing and consultation revealed deficits typical of the white matter dysfunction seen in MS. MRI scans showed new MS lesions affecting the white matter in multiple areas. She was started on immunomodulator treatment and remains on a proper schedule of routine neurologic care.

Unfortunately her cognitive problems, while not apparently worsening, were significant enough to preclude her from continuing in her profession, as she was unable to organize her daily classroom plan or keep track of different groups of children and activities occurring at the same time. The results of the neuropsychological consultation did allow for proper qualification for disability insurance and her retirement. She has the loving support of her husband and is doing well in other aspects of her life, including caring for her children and staying physically active.

A discussion of the state of her cognitive problems and performance is a continuing part of the assessment during her follow-up visits. Formal comparison of cognitive testing and consultation with the neuropsychologist will generally be a necessary part of long-term care in this scenario. Indeed, there are instances in the care of individuals when a worsening in cognitive function, compared with prior testing, is the motivating factor in making a decision to change immunomodulator therapy.

This is also when the observations by a spouse, significant other, family member, or friend can be critically important. Often a patient's spouse or friend can convey instances in which cognitive performance may be suspect. In converse, the spouse or friend may help to characterize events from another point of view, making it clear that the concerns of the patient are actually normal types of mental errors or forgetfulness. When cognitive deficits are present, it is important to try and have the spouse, family, and close friends aware and involved as much as it is appropriate for that individual.

Obviously, cognitive dysfunction may have an impact on the distribution of responsibilities in a family, on finances, and on other areas of social interaction both within and outside of a patient's immediate family. Sharing those concerns will serve to shift stressful responsibilities to the strength of others and save important cognitive energy for the patient.

There are also instances in which patients have specifically been referred for a cognitive decline due to MS. More commonly, there may be instances when, on an initial visit, a patient may raise a concern about a change in cognitive performance or question their memory or "speed of thinking." When cognition is part of the initial set of concerns in a patient with new or recently diagnosed MS, then early neuropsychological consultation should be obtained, and a discussion of these potential deficits and their importance is usually part of the first visit.

Scenario Three

On rare occasions, a patient may develop a specific type of cognitive deficit that can be attributed to a new active lesion also identified on MRI. A few notable patients come to mind, such as the interior designer who rather suddenly noted a vague sense that she could not recognize colleagues' faces. During a meeting, she had difficulty identifying colleagues with whom she regularly worked, until she heard their voices. For a number of days, she continued to sense a hesitation in perceiving facial features in a normal fashion. A new lesion was found in the temporal lobe of the brain in an area that could correlate with facial recognition. This problem in facial recognition resolved completely in a matter of a few weeks. We do continue to discuss this on some of her return visits to make sure that there has been no form of recurrence.

Another example is that of a college administrator who had the onset of mild difficulty in memory retrieval lasting a few days to a week. One evening, he was exercising and noticed the problem, and it became bad enough to prompt his family to take him to an emergency department. A thorough evaluation in the emergency department was unremarkable except for observing spotty difficulty in retrieving certain information on memory testing. He was not having difficulty making new memories or in concentration and attention. A brain MRI was performed, and a new active enhancing MS lesion was found in an area of the brain important in memory retrieval. These types of MS attacks that involve an isolated change in cognition due to a focal area of acute inflammation are unusual but need to be considered in the continuing care of patients with MS.

The important role that neuropsychologists have in the assessment and long-term care of people with MS cannot be overstated. Their research into MS cognitive deficits has provided the tools to detect and characterize these impairments, and their role in the routine care of MS patients is equally invaluable.

It is essential that neurologists involved in the care of patients with MS have access to excellent neuropsychologists comfortable and familiar with the illness and the type of cognitive deficits that may occur. Direct feedback from the neuropsychologist to the patient regarding interpretation of the test results and their meaning in context with the patient's symptoms and daily function can be critical. Definition of the character of any impairment that is discovered can help an individual understand the problem and create ideas to accommodate for it. Deficits discovered might help to justify a change in job or might be the principal factor deciding the outcome of disability adjudication.

I have seen a number of patients express relief that, despite the neuropsychologist having found an element of cognitive dysfunction attributable to their MS, they at least have an explanation and no longer think they are "going crazy." There have also been occasions when patients with a family history of Alzheimer disease were relieved to find out that the cognitive changes they were experiencing were clearly defined by the neuropsychologist as the type due to MS and not early Alzheimer disease.

Scenario Four

Another scenario worth mentioning has to do with the patient who has rather severe MS cognitive impairment. Although not common, in the most severe case, a patient's memory, concentration, processing speed, and other cognitive realms are so disrupted that the patients are completely dependent on others for their daily function and may require nearly constant around-the-clock care. Many times these individuals have poor insight into their deficits.

Other patients may clearly have moderate to severe deficits but might not acknowledge or realize this. I have seen patients with rather severe cognitive deficits who have continued to be employed, despite concerns of family and coworkers. Usually this is a job setting in which the duties and responsibilities are very routine or "overlearned," so that novel situations requiring learning or rapid decision making are not involved. On occasion, a patient must be directly confronted with the obvious impairment.

Most of the time, these individuals willingly accept the recommendation for further testing, counseling, and treatment; however, others may continue to deny that there is a problem. This can be difficult, especially if the person is unwilling to accept a recommendation for further testing or if there is no spouse or family to help intervene. Although the most severe degrees of cognitive impairment are not common, thankfully these patients usually welcome further evaluation and counseling, understand treatment recommendations, and have supportive family and friends. Additional support may be found through the local chapter of the National MS Society, government social service programs, and community- and church-based volunteer groups.

No matter our avocation, social situation, or background, our cognitive function is key to how we define ourselves and is critical in our ability to perform our various roles and meet our responsibilities. Attention to the potential deficits in cognitive function is an essential part of the standard of care for patients with MS. Neurologists should raise the subject for discussion at an appropriate time and be prepared to engage in ongoing dialogue about cognitive health. I realize that, in certain patients with no concerns regarding their cognition and no overt problems on their clinic visits, I may not directly ask about any perceived difficulties in their thinking as often as I intend. The patients should be informed in early discussions that it is an important subject and part of their continued care. Once the subject is brought out in the open, patients and their significant others should be made comfortable to report any cognitive concerns, including those that may seem trivial or simply normal behavior, on subsequent visits to their neurologist.

A valid consideration has been raised to include a neuropsychological consultation as part of a baseline evaluation in all people with MS, and assessment of cognitive function is now routinely a part of most clinical trials in MS treatment. Other trials of medication that may be helpful in improving cognition in MS are being undertaken. This further underscores how cognitive function has been properly included in the practical framework of current standard of care in MS. Now it is not uncommon for patients to bring up what they have read or heard regarding cognitive problems for further discussion during a clinic visit.

Neurologists need to directly include the discussion and assessment of cognitive function in their continuing care of patients with MS, and patients with MS should feel comfortable and encouraged to raise concerns or review persistent problems of cognition with their neurologists. This critical aspect of neurologic function must be considered a central element equal to all others in the comprehensive and compassionate care of people with MS. It is not acceptable to ignore the cognitive health concerns in MS. Patients should seek additional care if their questions regarding present or potential problems in their thinking are not being adequately addressed.

Mental Sharpening Stones and Perspectives

1. A direct discussion of cognitive performance should be a part of the ongoing assessment for patients with MS.
2. A review of specific aspects of cognitive performance allows a person to have more comfort in raising issues of concern and to distinguish normal behavior from possible problems due to their MS.
3. A potential change in cognition is as important as any other element of neurologic function threatened by MS, factoring into decisions on medical treatment.
4. A continued review of known specific areas of cognitive impairment should be part of routine neurologic follow-up visits.
5. When cognitive deficits are present, it is important for the family, spouse, significant others, and close friends to be aware of these problems and to be involved as much as is appropriate. This allows for a proper shift in stressful responsibilities onto those individuals and conserves vital cognitive energy for the patient.
6. An MS exacerbation may cause an isolated change in cognitive function due to a focal area of acute inflammation. This is not common but should not be overlooked as a diagnostic possibility in the continued evaluation of patients with MS.
7. It is essential that neurologists involved in the care of patients with MS have access to excellent neuropsychologists comfortable and familiar with the illness and the type of cognitive deficits that may occur.
8. Neurologists should raise the subject of the possible effect of MS on cognition for discussion at an appropri-

ate and early time and should be prepared to engage in an ongoing dialogue about cognitive health.

9. Patients and their significant others should be made comfortable to report and discuss any cognitive concerns.
10. If patient feels that their concerns regarding cognitive function are not being properly addressed or are uncomfortable discussing these concerns with their caregivers, then they should be encouraged to seek additional counsel from other neurologists, neuropsychologists, or allied healthcare support services for patients with MS.

Further Reading

Rao SM, Leo GJ, Bernardin L, Unverzagt F. Cognitive dysfunction in multiple sclerosis. I. Frequency, patterns, and prediction. *Neurology* 1991;41:685–691.

Heaton RK, Nelson LM, Thompson DS, Burks JS, Franklin GM. Neuropsychological findings in relapsing-remitting and chronic–progressive multiple sclerosis. *J Consult Clin Psychol* 1985; 53:103–110.

Bobholz JA, Rao SM. Cognitive dysfunction in multiple sclerosis. A review of recent developments. *Curr Opin Neurol* 2003; 6:283–288.

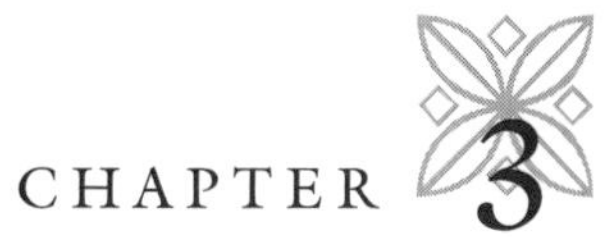

CHAPTER 3

My Mental Limp

Christy Demory

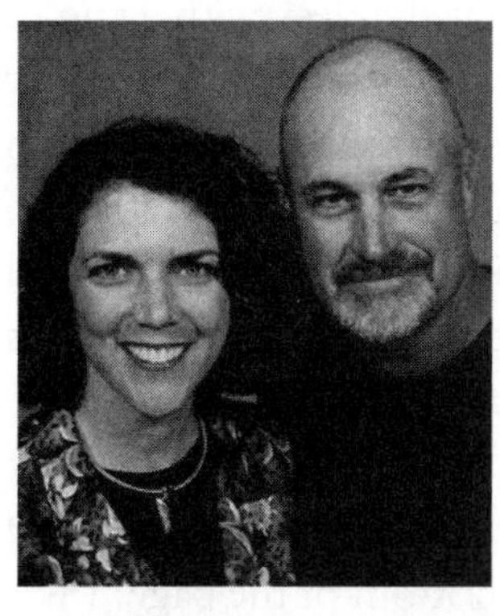

Ms. Demory is a retired U.S. Magistrate Judge who was compelled to leave the Federal bench due to the cognitive impairments from multiple sclerosis. Determined not to stay home, labeled as disabled, Ms. Demory decided to start her own business.

You can tell a lot about people by the way they respond to the inquiry, "Tell me a little bit about yourself." A few years ago, I would have said I was a partner in a large law firm with a litigation practice focused on complex commercial cases and construction disputes, with aspirations to become a judge. Today, I would say that I am happily married, have four girls (three canines and one feline), and teach women how to take care of their skin and project a professional image. A few years ago, if you would have told me that I would be a beauty consultant, I would have laughed in your face. Today, I can't imagine myself doing anything else.

So what prompted this transformation?

What could cause a person to jump ship at the height of a legal career and embrace in its stead the sale of lipstick? The cause was not readily identifiable. In fact, through various forms of disguise, it eluded recognition while it gradually permeated my mind. Literally. The cause is cognitive impairment resulting from multiple sclerosis (MS). Oh, I recognize it easily enough today, regardless of what name is used to identify it. Some prefer the phrase *cognitive challenges*; others prefer the term *neuropsychological deficits*. When I first confronted cognitive impairment a few years ago, I wasn't familiar with any of these terms or the havoc they can create.

My relationship with cognitive issues began shortly after I was diagnosed with MS. A vivid memory of that day remains. An episode of vertigo, facial paralysis, and hearing loss kept me out of work for six weeks. After a healthy course of IV steroids, the vertigo and paralysis were gone, my hearing had returned, and I was ready to get back to work. Sitting down at my desk with a cup of coffee, I tried to jump back in where I had left off. The first order of business was to get caught up in all my cases. A memorandum of law lay innocently on my desk. With eagerness I picked it up and began to read. I reread and reheated my coffee, and read again. A few hours later, I walked next door to my partner's office, closed the door, and buried my head in my hands.

"I've lost it," I cried. There was no comprehension of what I had been reading for hours. My mind couldn't carry the thread of thought from the top of the page to the bottom of the page. I was physically and mentally exhausted. Frustrated and defeated, I went home to rest, hoping that things would be better the next day.

Throughout the next several weeks, this pattern continued and my frustration grew. Never before had I had difficulty with comprehension or concentration. Suddenly, it seemed, I couldn't keep my mind focused. I had never heard of cognitive impairments and made no connection between what I was experiencing and my recent MS diagnosis. Perhaps my mind was distracted, or preoccupied, or both. After all, I recently had become engaged, was planning a wedding, and had just been told that I had an incurable disease of the central nervous system. Being 36 and childless, my biologic clock was ticking. Not enough? Well, I also was dealing with the realization that, in my effort to build a successful legal career, I had failed to build a life. That hurt.

Yes, I had good reason to be distracted, but, let's face it, this wasn't the first time that I had had a full plate of worries. Work always had been the tool that enabled me to deal with the "stuff" of life. My brother was killed in a tragic accident—I worked through it. My parents went through a painful divorce—I worked through it. There were times of loneliness and emptiness—I worked through that, too. Never before had I experienced such difficulty concentrating. No, this time it was different. The more I tried to work, the less I accomplished, and my frustration grew. Not knowing what else to do, I continued to keep myself busy at work but found myself gravitating toward those tasks that were more administrative and ministerial, rather than analytical.

Exhaustion was now a part of my life. Complete physical and mental exhaustion. Sometimes, the fatigue was so overwhelming that it was a struggle to stay alert and awake while at work. I couldn't wait to return to my neurologist for the first of many follow-up appointments. When I told my doctor about the difficulty I was having with concentration and focus, he prescribed Prozac.

"Oh great," I thought, "He thinks I'm depressed." Was I depressed? I certainly didn't feel depressed, and my life was getting back on track. I was feeling much better and my physical symptoms had subsided. It took a year before I was willing to admit to my depression. My doctor said that the Prozac would help with the concentration and the fatigue, so I swallowed the pills and continued to do the only thing I knew to do: work. When starting my day earlier to maximize the morning hours didn't help, I flipped it around and tried working later in the day. When it came to reading, my finger became a guide to help keep me focused on the page. Large documents were broken down into small subparts, sometimes by paragraph, so that I could absorb them bit by bit. And as I experimented with my work schedule, the fatigue continued, and exercise became more and more difficult.

My law practice continued while an internal struggle ensued. Was I trying hard enough or, perhaps, trying too hard? Was I still a good lawyer or was I ever a good lawyer? Would the passion and zeal for my work return? Had I really "lost it?" As questions such as these swarmed through my mind, there was the ever-present stress in a large-firm litigation practice. Billable hours. Court schedules and deadlines. All of these things made me wonder if I could ever again be truly effective as a lawyer. It wasn't that I couldn't figure things out. No, my IQ hadn't changed. My intelligence, education, and experience were still intact. I just had to work harder mentally to find answers, to solve problems, and to put the pieces together.

This extra mental effort left me exhausted and spent at the end of the day. My frustration was compounded by the fact that no one could see the difficulty I was having. It was all in my head—literally. There were no visible physical signs of my struggle. I remember walking my dog one morning, feeling sorry for myself, and wishing in some distorted way that I had a limp or some other physical manifestation that I could point to and say, "See, that's why I'm so tired."

That's when I realized that I did in fact have a limp—a *mental limp*. I thought with an invisible limp. Although I was still able to go through the mental rigors of analysis and problem solving, it simply took me longer to get to the end point, just like it takes a person with a physical limp longer to walk from one end of the room to the other.

A picture that is often seen on greeting cards depicts a cat hanging from a tree branch in chin-up position accompanied by the caption, "Hang in there, baby!" This picture appropriately describes my professional life during the months that followed. My work consisted largely of hanging on and not letting anything slip through the cracks, while I struggled with my mental limp and related fatigue. As a litigator, my work revolved around problems. Either a client had been sued and, therefore, wasn't happy, or a client had been wronged and, therefore, wasn't happy. Whichever the case, it was my responsibility to navigate the sometimes tumultuous waters of the adversarial process and work out an acceptable resolution.

Handling several cases at a time was a challenge, each with its own unique circumstances and deadlines. Twelve-and 14-hour days at the office were the norm. Even when I wasn't physically at the office, there were many times that I was mentally there, mulling over situations, thinking through problems. My mind got little opportunity to truly rest, and my stamina waned. Whereas I used to spend hours reading and researching, these tasks now left me exhausted. When the fatigue would set in, no amount of effort on my part could resist its influence. The sleep that would overtake me was not the peaceful kind, but the insistent and unrelenting kind. Fatigue became my tireless and unwavering enemy.

As the months rolled on and my mental limping continued, I quickly realized that I needed to reduce both the level of stress in my life and the number of hours I worked. I didn't know how I could do this and continue my law practice, so I decided to resign from private practice and take a job as a staff attorney for the United States District Court. My job was to review appeals by state death-row inmates. The court records in such cases are voluminous and the issues of the utmost significance. In spite of the heaviness of the work, both emotionally and analytically, the job did not involve the stresses and pressures of a private law practice, and it seemed the perfect opportunity. The transition was smooth. Since I was working fewer hours, I was able to focus on developing some healthy habits and giving my mind and body adequate rest. There even was time for relaxing with friends and family, playing a round of golf, and singing in my church choir.

Although I was feeling good physically, the cognitive challenges continued to come and go. At times, my concentration and problem-solving skills were cooperative and my work flowed smoothly. At others, concentration was a laborious task that quickly led to exhaustion. I began battling severe excessive daytime fatigue. My office phone would ring, breaking the silence with the startling realization that I had fallen asleep. Sometimes, I would awaken and find myself slumped over my desk, my work papers spread out underneath me. On bad days, my mind's urgent demand for sleep was quite predictable—you could almost set your clock by it. Nothing I did deterred it. Medication brought some temporary improvement in my alertness, but the side-effects were bothersome and interfered with my normal sleep, so I discontinued its use.

Through all of this, my frustration with myself increased. Was I just not trying hard enough? Did I need to get more sleep at night? It was very difficult to explain my struggles, especially when I "looked so good." My *mental limp* was no longer an adequate explanation, and I had no believable way to describe the extreme fatigue that overtook me on a daily basis. This cycle of fatigue and mental lethargy led me to my first coping strategy.

Know Your Body's Rhythm

Of course, I didn't identify it as a strategy at the time, since my primary concern was professional survival. I discovered that certain activities and tasks brought on the fatigue more readily than others. Tasks such as reading and analyzing made me very susceptible to the fatigue, whereas other tasks, such as organizing documents or discussing issues with others, never seemed to drain me. It became clear to me that there were predictably "good" times and "bad" times throughout the day.

The morning hours generally were the most productive for me. My concentration and focus during the morning hours were not impaired, and I could read for long periods without falling asleep. My lapses in concentration and fatigue typically would strike in the early afternoon. Almost without exception, my afternoon attempts to read and concentrate were rewarded with nothing more than a deep sleep. Even when I was successful in staying awake, mental acuity still eluded me. Like a lens out of focus, my thoughts seemed unable to converge to yield a lucid idea.

It became obvious to me that I needed to avoid intense cognitive tasks in the afternoon. I wasn't physically tired at that time of day, nor was my physical energy lacking. My mind was simply exhausted, and I didn't completely understand what was happening. It was clear to me that, if I was left alone to read or engage in other intense cognitive tasks, it would only be a matter of time before the uncontrollable and overwhelming need to sleep would overtake me. My situation was much like that of a deep-sea diver, whose length of time underwater is determined by the depth of the dive. The deeper one goes, the shorter the dive must be, lest the diver's air supply be exhausted. For me, the duration of my cognitive stamina—my air supply— was directly controlled by the intensity of my cognitive demands.

Plan Your Activities According to Your Body's Rhythm

When I made the connection between my activities and my energy level, I started scheduling the tasks that required cognitive skills for my peak energy times, to get the most out of my performance. For example, since I was most alert during the morning hours, I would try to get most of my reading, analysis, and intense concentration done during these hours. If I was on a roll and making strides, I wouldn't even answer the phone. After all, I had voice mail and could respond to questions during the afternoon hours. Conferences and meetings were scheduled for the afternoon hours as well, as were the tasks that were more administrative, such as organizing documents and preparing reports. Even as I've been writing this chapter, my morning hours have been the most productive. (Oh, the times that I had a great thought developing, only to find myself sound asleep, head rolled to the side, laptop perched on my lap, fingers still on the keyboard!)

Understand the Nature of Your Cognitive Limitations

As my mental limping continued, I began looking for answers. Common sense told me that I needed to educate myself about MS cognitive issues. Not knowing where else to turn, I started with the internet. Reliable websites such as that of the National Multiple Sclerosis Society provided helpful information about cognitive issues. I scoured publications such as *InsideMS* and *MSFocus* for any mention of cognitive problems. Whenever I had the opportunity, I talked to others with MS to see if they shared my experiences with cognitive challenges and fatigue. The more I learned about cognitive issues, the more convinced I became that what I was experiencing was real.

The idea of neuropsychological testing was planted by a friend who has MS, whose neurologist had requested it for her. She explained the testing to me, how it could measure cognitive abilities and be used as a baseline to evaluate future performance. I wanted this, too. I needed to know whether it was all in my head (no pun intended). To measure future cognitive changes, I would need this testing as a baseline.

The long and arduous testing was administered by a neuropsychologist. When it was all said and done, I felt like an abysmal failure. When she sat down with me to explain the findings, it was most helpful and enlightening. Although my IQ and general pool of knowledge were intact, my mental processing speed was slow, and I had reduced stamina in responding to visual stimuli. Aha! This explained why my concentration and focus would fade and I often fell asleep while reading lengthy documents. In contrast, I performed better in response to audio stimuli, which explained why I could discuss issues and process through issues with others without becoming fatigued. As crazy as all of this sounded at first, it made perfect sense to me. It also explained why it was taking me longer to wrap my mind around issues.

Armed with some objective data, I discussed my situation with my employer and shared my concerns. Up to this point, my only solution for my *mental limp* was to take vacation or sick leave when a 40-hour week was too much for me. Not surprisingly, my vacation and sick leave had been exhausted quickly and I needed another solution. My employer was very understanding and allowed me to take leave without pay when I needed to rest. At least I wouldn't have to feel guilty about sleeping on the job!

For the first time since my cognitive symptoms surfaced, I saw a ray of hope. My flexible work schedule was working well for me. It enabled me to work hard when I could and to rest as needed. Since I had invested the time and resources to identify my weaknesses and understand my cognitive impairments, I was able to adapt my work to maximize my effectiveness. My mornings were reserved for reading, and long documents were broken down into manageable segments. After reading a segment, I would write a short synopsis and then take a short break before continuing. During the afternoon hours, I scheduled time to discuss and debate issues with my colleagues. Yes, I scheduled time to give my mind a rest.

As my sense of worth returned, so did my passion and zeal for my profession. When a position became available in the court for a part-time magistrate judge, I applied. A part-time schedule, it seemed, would be perfect for me. And the work would be varied, challenging, and rewarding!

On May 3, 2004, I was sworn in as a United States Magistrate Judge, serving in a part-time capacity. My professional dream was fulfilled! I embraced my new duties and responsibilities with fervor and excitement and took very seriously my oath to protect and defend the Constitution of the United States. In criminal proceedings, my duties included conducting initial appearances and detention hearings in which a decision in most instances had to be made expeditiously and on the spot. My auditory attention was not impaired, and I thrived in the courtroom, listening to arguments, applying the law to the facts before me, and striving to provide justice.

When I wasn't in the courtroom, I was in chambers, where I was immersed in a civil caseload of social security appeals. The work involved reading, research, analysis, and decision making. Since I was not working a full-time schedule, I was able to rest when I needed. However, I soon discovered a new devil with which I had to contend: interruptions! A magistrate judge's authority includes the issuance of search warrants and arrest warrants. These matters often come before the court with a sense of urgency and must be handled expediently. It was not unusual during my day to receive phone calls or visits from law enforcement officers requesting the issuance of a warrant. In addition, I received regular communication from court personnel regarding upcoming matters and scheduling issues.

Over time, it became increasingly difficult to recapture my train of thought on a matter after an interruption. Hours of reading, research, and analysis would be lost after having to redirect my attention to a more exigent matter. Working within the confines of a part-time schedule, I did my best to manage my varied judicial responsibilities and minimize interruptions, but the judicial process cannot always be planned and scheduled. Eventually, the time came when greater efficiency was demanded of me in the one area that was my weakest: the reading, research, and analysis in my civil caseload. When it became clear that the expectations regarding the quantity of work produced were greater than I could perform, it was agreed that I would step down from my position.

To say that this was a difficult decision is an understatement. So much of my identity as a person had been wrapped up in my professional status. Not only did stepping down from my judicial position signal the end of my legal career, it suggested that MS had won the battle that I had fought for so long. I had failed. Notwithstanding what appeared to be the best of circumstances—a part-time judicial position—my cognitive capacities were not cooperating. Accepting this fate was not easy, but I needed to embrace the fact that who I was as a person was not dependent on my profession.

My heart told me that I still had much to contribute to my community, and while I refused to simply quit on myself and do nothing, what would I do? The answer came in a most unexpected way: through a bottle of moisturizer. Although Mary Kay was a household name, it was one I associated with pink cars and big hair. However, I had started using the products a few years earlier and loved them. Sensing my frustration with my career, my friend and beauty consultant shared with me about the career opportunity.

By sharing Mary Kay skin care and cosmetic products with other women and teaching them how to take care of their skin, I would have the opportunity to generate product sales and build a customer base that would provide a steady flow of income through reorders. This was unfamiliar territory for me, as I knew nothing about skin care and wore very little makeup, but my friend would be available to provide hands-on training opportunities. Additional training would be available through audiovisual materials, manuals, and the internet, all of which could be used at my own pace. There were no sales quotas and I could set my own hours, work as much or as little as I wanted, and choose the type of appointments to hold.

This all sounded good to me, but I was resistant at first. After all, I had worked very hard to develop my legal career and had a hard time seeing myself as a lipstick lady. The more I learned about the career opportunities in Mary Kay, the company, and its founder, Mary Kay Ash, the more convinced I became that this could be a viable career opportunity for me. After all, the role of beauty consultant did not require the intense rigors of research, reading, and analysis that were part of my legal work. If I found ways to work in my cognitive strengths and minimize the time working in my cognitive weaknesses, then I could make this work.

The prospect of launching out on my own and helping other women feel good about themselves intrigued me. My role essentially would be that of a teacher, something I knew I could and would love to do. In fact, my very first job was that of a teacher—teaching piano at the ripe age of 13. Since that time, my teaching experience has covered a wide array of subjects, from piano and aerobic exercise, to computerized legal research and public speaking. Teaching women about their skin would just be another subject that I knew I could learn.

Opening a business was a new experience for me, as was running one on a day-to-day basis. Not surprisingly, some people around me thought I had really lost my mind! They questioned why I would want to assume the responsibility of a business while dealing with MS and, particularly, the fatigue I was experiencing. What my well-meaning friends and family didn't realize was that the work I engaged in to build my business actually replenished my energy, rather than depleted it. I was not venturing out solo into uncharted waters, since my friend who introduced me to the career had promised to guide me. The company itself had a wealth of training materials.

My first assignment in my new business was to contact everyone I knew and ask for their help in getting started. Friends generally are a supportive and understanding audience. Mine were eager to let me sit down with them and share my budding knowledge of skin care, while allowing them to try some new products. At the same time, my networking skills were being developed. I began asking for referrals. Soon, my friends and customers were introducing me to their friends. This enabled me to build a large customer base and a reservoir of contacts to make sure there always were appointments to hold. However, the development of a large customer and referral base created the need for another cognitive strategy.

Develop a Reliable Method to Handle Important Information

For me, the important information that I must manage includes contact information about referrals and prospective customers. Many well-intentioned friends and customers would pass along referrals in a very haphazard fashion. Sometimes, it was a comment made in passing during an unrelated conversation. Many times, it would be through the transfer of a miscellaneous piece of paper: the back of a receipt, a gum wrapper, a corner torn from a sheet of paper. These random pieces of paper quickly became unmanageable, and some pieces even were lost. Frequently, when the slip of paper contained just a name and number, I was unable to recall who had given me the name. I needed a system to organize and maintain these referrals.

In order to bring some uniformity and manageability to my referrals, I started using an index card system. Whenever a referral is given to me, I record the pertinent information—name, phone number, email, person making the referral, and date the referral was made—on an index card. Then, I sort the cards in two groups. The first group represents those I have made an attempt to contact, and they are stored alphabetically. The second group represents those I have not yet contacted, and they are stored chronologically.

Managing referral information is simply one example of information that needs to be managed. One thing is certain: if you are reading this chapter, then you have information to manage. It may be as mundane as paying bills or something complex related to your work. By developing a system to effectively manage the information that you need, your cognitive energy will be preserved for more demanding or challenging tasks.

Identify and Perpetuate the Activities That Maximize Your Cognitive Strengths

As I began working in my new business and holding appointments with customers, I discovered a renewed source of energy. Regardless of the time of day, teaching a skin-care class filled me with energy. The more time I spent interacting with others, the more energy I seemed to have. These activities employed auditory skills that, as reflected in the results of my neuropsychological testing, were not impaired. These activities also did not require intense cognitive processing of information. The more that I worked in the areas of my cognitive strengths, the more energy I had—both mental and physical.

Knowing this, I schedule time each day to focus on activities that utilize my areas of strength. I focus on personal contacts, either in person or on the phone, and look for opportunities to teach and to be with my customers. When I'm not with my customers, I'm looking for opportunities to train other consultants. Personal interaction with others is crucial. Not surprisingly, when I do this, I experience much less daytime drowsiness and excessive thinking fatigue!

Identify and Limit the Activities That Exploit Your Weaknesses

This strategy naturally follows from knowing your strengths. When we understand our weaknesses, we can plan our work accordingly. For example, written communication, which involves visual attention and stamina, is one of my weaknesses. However, occasional note writing is necessary. My note-writing activities are scheduled for my peak cognitive time or in small increments during other activities in which plenty of auditory stimuli are available.

Another area of weakness for me relates to memory. It can be difficult to retain important information or keep up with multiple things at the same time. My unreliable memory and slow speed of processing information made it difficult for me to keep track of details. Handling multiple tasks simultaneously was exhausting. These are weaknesses that needed to be managed. On more than one occasion, I missed meetings or appointments because I forgot to write them down on my calendar. On one occasion, I arrived for an appointment at the wrong time. This was not tardiness. It was forgetting that the appointment had been reset for 4:00, not 6:00. With repeated failures of this nature, it was tempting to give up and feel sorry for myself, but I wanted to succeed. Clearly, I wasn't the first person to ever deal with cognitive challenges.

It would be appropriate at this point to restate the obvious. Everything in my new career has not gone smoothly. There have been many mistakes. I've mixed up customer orders, forgotten about orders, and even forgotten about appointments! When talking about coping strategies, I believe that the discussion actually should begin with the premise that we—those of us dealing with MS cognitive challenges—must have the desire and determination to overcome them. Patience is required, as is the willingness to make some mistakes. Each of us faces a unique set of circumstances. What has worked for you may not work for me, and vice versa. It's through my mistakes that I have learned what will and will not work for me. No doubt, the same is true for you.

Dr. John C. Maxwell wrote a book entitled *Failing Forward*, which helped me understand this concept. If we are not willing to risk failure, then we will never find what works for us. The coping strategies that I have embraced were developed through this long and sometimes arduous process of failing forward.

Create Safety Nets to Reinforce Areas of Cognitive Weakness

Safety nets provide reinforcement and confidence in those areas impacted by our cognitive weaknesses. First, we must understand our areas of weakness and how they impact our activities before we can make accommodations to minimize their effect on our day-to-day functioning. It was evident from the start that my memory impairment affected my ability to run my business. One of the first safety nets I developed was a system to prevent oversights and poor customer service on my part. I needed to develop a planning system that would help me manage my schedule and record my daily activities with efficiency. I toyed with several different types of planning and calendar systems, trying to find one that would work for me.

First, I tried a handheld personal data assistant to keep my calendar and customer information. This was a helpful and efficient tool, but, because of its compact size, it was frequently missing in action—or perhaps it was my memory that was MIA. Regardless, I was constantly losing it. Moreover, customer information was often missing, primarily due to my failure to update or synchronize the handheld device with my computer, where information was input and stored. A few missed appointments and misdirected customer orders made me realize that I needed another system.

The planning system that I currently use includes a date book and a "brain" book. My date book consists of both a monthly and a weekly calendar. The monthly calendar is used to schedule appointments and plan events. It shows me the big picture. The weekly calendar serves as my daily guide. Once a week, I sit down with my monthly calendar and my weekly calendar and plan my week. I choose to do my weekly planning on Sunday evening, when I am relaxed and refreshed. This also gives me a smooth transition from the end of the weekend to the start of a new week.

The appointments for the week that are set on the monthly calendar are transferred to the weekly calendar. Once my appointments are in place, other activities and errands are scheduled. Ideally, my other activities and errands, such as going to the dry cleaners and trips to the post office, are coordinated around my appointments to make efficient use of my travel time. Once that is completed, my focus shifts to the personal priorities that I want to complete for the week. I schedule my exercise time and visits with family and friends. Even a date night with my husband is scheduled. My goal is to have my entire week, from business appointments to personal massages, mapped out on my weekly calendar. When Monday morning arrives, my direction is clear, and I don't have to expend mental energy to figure out what I'm supposed to be doing, and when.

This system also helps me see when I'm trying to be too much of an overachiever. When my weekly calendar is booked solid from morning to night, with no scheduled breaks, that's a clue that I need to either delegate or hire help. As you might imagine, this system does take time. Typically, I spend between 30 and 45 minutes each Sunday evening just planning out my week, but it is time well spent. Every minute spent in planning pays off exponentially in execution. This system was cumbersome and awkward at first but is easily perfected through practice and repetition. Today, I can't imagine doing without my weekly calendar.

The second part of my planning system is what I call my "brain" book. To the untrained eye, it looks like an ordinary spiral notebook. To me, it's another safety net. Since memory is a problem for me, I write down everything that needs to be remembered in my brain book. I start a fresh notebook every month, so the 70-page notebooks are efficient and not too cumbersome. The brain book is my constant companion, going everywhere with me. It is the chronologic record of my days. Its pages contain notes from every phone call, contact or referral, voicemail message, meeting or consultation, expenses, and every random thought that darts through my mind that I want to remember.

Basically, if I need to remember it, it goes in the brain book. If it's something that requires follow-up or future action, it goes in the brain book. In fact, if my brain book is not accessible when an important thought comes along, I'll call my voice mail and leave the details in a message to myself. Since my voice mail messages are recorded in my brain book, this ensures that the thought will not be lost or forgotten. This is incredibly liberating, knowing that I don't have to try to "hold on" to a thought until it can be appropriately written down. It preserves my mental energy for more important tasks.

As the month progresses, my brain book serves as the transcript of my days. Like any other record, it can be reviewed as needed. At the end of each week, I go back through my brain book to make sure there's nothing left undone. Were all phone calls returned, voice mail messages appropriately handled, and all product deliveries made? In essence, it serves as a *safety net* to ensure that everything that needed to get done was completed. If not, then the oversight is discovered in a timely fashion and corrective action can be self-initiated. I would much prefer to call my customer to let her know that I forgot to mail her order, rather than to have the customer call me wondering where it was! At the end of the month, the review process is repeated for the entire month's notes just to make sure nothing was left undone. Once everything is completed, the month's brain book is filed away and a new one is started.

The brain book system was not my idea but was suggested by a friend who was tired of hearing me complain about forgetting things and hearing my frustration when I forgot customer orders and appointments. Her interest in helping me find a solution escalated the day I forgot to meet her for lunch. Fortunately, she was quick to forgive. The primary advantage of my brain book system is that it takes away the worry and stress—the mental weight—of "I have to remember this!" The presence of a reliable memory safety net gives me peace of mind.

The use of the computer also can be a great cognitive safety net. For those of us with cognitive challenges, the computer can work for us in our areas of weakness. The use of a computer is essential to the management of my business, particularly in managing important information and keeping track of commitments. I sought out the resources and technical tools that not only would serve the needs of my business, but also would make up for my cognitive weaknesses. To begin my research, I spoke with other beauty consultants about their use of the computer, the software programs used, and how the computer was integrated into their businesses. Software vendors also were willing to share their suggestions and ideas. As a result, my computer literacy and proficiency have greatly improved over the past few years. Before starting my business, my computer skills were limited to using basic word-processing software, checking email, and searching the internet. Now I use databases and spreadsheets, inventory management software, and financial management software. I'm living proof that even the cognitively impaired can learn computer skills.

The business management software program I utilize was recommended to me by a friend. This software program stores customer sales, expenses, and customer data, such as personal contact information, birthday and anniversary, product preferences, and order histories. It also allows me to maintain an annotated log of all my customer contacts. Where my own memory is fickle, my computer is reliable. In essence, the computer serves as my surrogate memory!

In case you're wondering why I keep a customer contact log on the computer when I have my brain book, let me explain the difference in the two. The brain book is a working document that gets me through each month. It is not designed to track long-range tasks and follow-up activities. At the end of the month, it has served its purpose and is filed away. On the other hand, the computer allows me to specify a follow-up date at any time in the future.

The computer also is a great communication tool that can "hide" our good and bad times throughout the day. Since e-mail does not require an immediate response, I can schedule time to respond to e-mail when I am energized and refreshed. Some customers prefer to be contacted via e-mail. With a quick e-mail, I can see how they're doing, find out if they need anything, and let them know about new products and specials that may be of interest to them. My personal website is a safety net where my customers can contact me and shop 24/7. This was actually a very easy decision and required no technical knowledge or skill on my part, since it is maintained by Mary Kay, Inc. For a nominal annual fee, the company updates the site, personalizes it for me, and handles all the technical aspects.

The first strategy I identified, knowing your body's rhythm, is also very important in my business. I schedule the non-people–related tasks, such as logging expenses, writing notes, and studying about new products, for the mornings when I am at my cognitive peak. Time spent with people energizes and refreshes me, so most of my people time takes place in the afternoon and early evening. Knowing your body's good and bad times is crucial to being able to schedule your tasks in a way that maximizes your effectiveness and efficiency.

Find a Mentor

Most of the strategies I've discussed have involved individual effort. We each must take a certain amount of personal responsibility to overcome the obstacles and challenges that we face. However, this is not to minimize the benefit of having others around you to whom you can be accountable. A mentor is someone who can provide guidance, direction, and feedback in an area, based upon her or his own experience and expertise in that area. Honestly, it's difficult for me to be objective about my challenges and obstacles. I get so wrapped up in the "whine" of my failures—"I can't get it all done!" or "I can't remember things!" When my brain is limping and I can't concentrate that hard—I can't see the why.

A good mentor can help you identify the "why" behind your obstacles or struggles. Often, the reason we don't see the why ourselves is because we are too close to the problem. The mentor looks over the situation with a broader, more distanced perspective and objectivity that enables her to identify not only the reason for the problems, but also potential solutions. A mentor with experience in your problem area or your business field can guide you to strategies for coping and managing the problems.

When I was having difficulty setting priorities between personal health issues and business goals, the mentor I enrolled was a woman who, while battling cancer for more than 20 years, had built a multimillion dollar business. Through her experiences, she was able to help me sort through these seemingly competing priorities and achieve a productive balance. Similarly, it was a mentor who managed a busy household with four school-aged children, while she was building a successful business, who suggested I keep a brain book and review it weekly and monthly.

My mentors have varied over time, from others in my own business organization who are at a level where I want to be, to persons in other professions who have overcome similar obstacles. Accountability requires a degree of vulnerability, which can be uncomfortable, mainly because we are making our weaknesses public. A true mentor will not take advantage of this position of trust. A true mentor recognizes that we all need help, at times. In order for a mentor relationship to be most effective, it's important that the relationship be established before problems occur. Think of the mentor relationship as preventive medicine—an objective assessment of your systems and strategies.

Recognize That You Don't Have to Do Everything

As I worked through my cognitive struggles, I found myself taking on more and more responsibilities in my business. If something needed to be done, then I assumed I needed to do it. After all, it was my business and I wanted to prove to myself, and perhaps to others, that I could handle it all. Well, that's a mistake. The more effort I expended on tasks that were not in my strengths, the less effective I was in my other work. In essence, I was spending dollar time on penny tasks and using up my limited cognitive reservoir on activities that were not that important. By delegating the tasks that either drain me or don't maximize my strengths, I am freed up to focus on what is most important for my business and my productivity.

This endeavor has brought some unexpected benefits as well. My people skills, which were never very good, have developed and have become a great asset in my business. Working with my customers is very rewarding and enables me to walk beside them through their own periods of joy and sorrow. My customers and business associates have become wonderful friends. They have taught me the value of good relationships and have shown me the joy and fulfillment that come from being able to care for, encourage, and inspire others.

As I share my knowledge of skin care with my customers, I also share my own MS journey. This has given me the opportunity to share some of the lessons I've learned. The lessons I've learned about being true to my values and setting priorities that embrace those values, about the importance of treasuring each and every day, about making a positive attitude a matter of choice, not chance. MS taught me that my success was not defined by what I received from the world, but by what I gave to the world. It taught me to laugh and enjoy this ride around the sun and, yes, even to laugh at myself.

My work, now, is work of the heart. Mary Kay teaches that we should imagine everyone we meet with an invisible sign around their neck that reads "make me feel important." That's my goal. Whether it's taking the time to smile at the store clerk who's obviously having a bad day or sending a card to a customer for no reason other than to say "I'm thinking of you," my new career gives the freedom and flexibility to really focus on others. Not surprisingly, because I am no longer burdened by the cognitive rigors of research and analysis that were an integral part of my legal work, my cognitive and physical fatigue have drastically diminished.

My journey with cognitive challenges has been an enlightening one. I've had to let go of a legal career and embrace a new career selling cosmetics. My understanding of success has changed. It is no longer based on outward things such as a salary, title, or position. Instead, success for me is found in doing my best each and every day, living each day without regrets, and being a bright spot in someone else's day. It has been, and continues to be, a rewarding journey. There is much more that I intend to do and I am far from being done. My cognitive coping strategies no doubt will need to be revisited and revised from time to time. That is part of the process of growth and change.

And as you continue your journey, I hope that these strategies will serve you, too, and propel you forward in your journey. The strategies shared in these pages took years to develop and refine. They required a certain degree of flexibility and daringness. Don't be afraid to try new things and fail forward. Certainly, don't be afraid to build upon the strategies I have shared. Embrace what works for you, and discard what doesn't. Make modifications and adjustments where you find it necessary to make your own strategies that will work for you. But never give up. Discover what's around the next corner.

Mental Sharpening Stones and Perspectives

1. Know your body's rhythm and the predictably good and bad functioning times throughout the day.
2. Plan your activities and tasks according to your body's rhythm, and schedule intense cognitive tasks for your peak times.
3. Understand that your intelligence, education, and experience remain intact; cognitive impairments just require that we adapt how we function and employ them.

4. Understand the nature of your cognitive limitations.
5. Identify the activities that exploit your cognitive strengths and energize you, and schedule these activities on a regular basis.
6. Identify the tasks and activities that are impacted by your cognitive weaknesses, and schedule these activities during peak times.
7. Be patient with yourself; let go of perfectionism and be willing to make mistakes along the way. The trial-and-error method will pay off in the end.
8. Create safety nets to reinforce your areas of weakness and redirect your cognitive energies to productive tasks.
9. Don't put undue pressure on yourself to remember everything; develop a reliable safety net for your memory.
10. Create systems to effectively handle data and relieve the unnecessary cognitive drain of storing and recalling information.
11. Find a good mentor or accountability partner with whom you can share ideas, receive honest feedback, and accept encouragement and advice.
12. Don't try to do it all; delegate as much as you can so that your cognitive energies are reserved for those tasks that truly must be done by you.
13. Recognize that life is precious and each moment counts.

CHAPTER 4

Popping the Clutch

Dan Waters

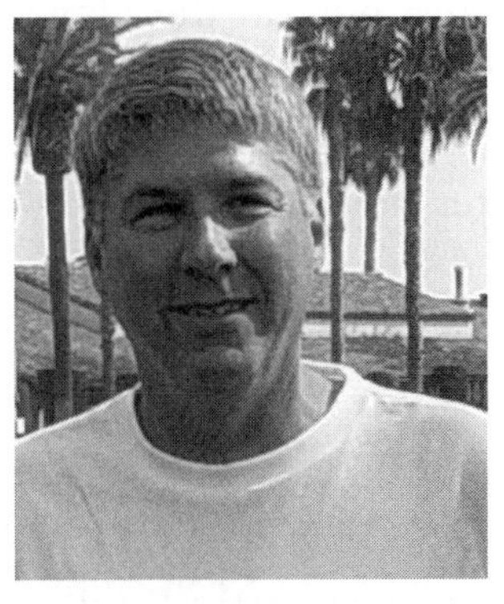

Daniel W. Waters enjoyed a 10-year career in the United States Marine Corps. After his honorable discharge, he began a successful and rewarding career in manufacturing, first as a buyer, then as a sales engineer, and finally as president and owner of an industry-leading executive recruiting business. Dan was diagnosed with multiple sclerosis in 2005.

When I was teenager, I had the pride and pleasure of buzzing around in my father's red 1964 Ford dump truck. Compared to today's large (quads), it was a smaller, yard-scape type with dualies and four-wheel drive. The truck had no starter, so this meant that we strategically parked the truck on hills before shutting it off. This way, when I released the brake, the truck would begin rolling down hill, and I could pop the clutch to get it started again. I loved this little truck and have many fond teenage memories and experiences.

Janice, a vibrant, fun young lady was the first girl I dated. I still remember her bewildered look while driving around the movie theater, searching for the "right" place to park. Each time we circled the lot, we moved further from the theater to find a hill and would park. The cold winter walk back to the theater was five blocks, and the next day at school, everyone knew why I had made Janice walk!

It wasn't long after my first dating experience that a beautiful young girl named Kathy moved from Milwaukee to Kettle Moraine. She knew nothing of my father's little red truck and agreed to go out on a date! She seemed to not mind the walk. In fact, we talked while we walked, and, to this day, the connection is strong—soul mates for sure. Kathy, an adventurous young lady, and I, carefree and wild, were a match made in heaven! Five years later, we married and Janice was the bridesmaid.

Immediately after the wedding, I took Kathy on a honeymoon that would last seven years and include places like Cherry Point, North Carolina; Iwakuni, Japan; and Tustin, California. Having already served three years of active duty in the United States Marine Corps, I was convinced that we were ready to see the world and experience the military lifestyle together and whatever other adventures we would encounter along the way.

Acceleration

Early in my career, I spent a year overseas stationed on Okinawa, Japan, a beautiful island located between mainland Japan and Taiwan. I loved the plush mountainous scenery, the Asian culture, and especially the scuba diving, as this area of the globe was considered to be among the very best in the world. A few of us would frequently skin dive at night for octopus, a Japanese delicacy, and, when steamed, is something I still enjoy while dining in a traditional Japanese restaurant. During that year of duty, I began having annoying discomfort in both of my knees, which in time escalated to pain and, then, barely tolerable pain. Tylenol, Advil, Motrin, taken three at a time, several times daily, gave no real relief. With frequent visits to sick bay, I was diagnosed with chondromalacia, a degeneration of cartilage in the knee, usually caused by excessive wear between the patella and lower end of the femur.

It was thought to be caused by running, perhaps excessive running in combat boots, and I was instructed to not run for a while.

A couple of months later, a few of us gathered for dinner at our favorite place for chicken fried rice. Somehow, on this one particular night, I was just not feeling right. I was somewhat dizzy, seeing double, and my speech had become slightly slurred. Cupping my hand over my left eye, I continued to sip hot tea while being thankful that our dinner was short. Normally, the mile walk back to base would take 10 or 15 minutes, only this time it seemed to take an eternity. I was being assisted by two fellow Marines, with the world spinning as I struggled to walk. All I could think about was "what is wrong" and "get me to my rack." Once there, I stayed and rested until midafternoon the next day. Completely weak with exhaustion, I stumbled to sick bay and, because I had no temperature, vomiting, or congestion, I was given Tylenol and bed rest. It was thought to be some sort of virus, so I was told.

Everything I needed to know about being a Marine I learned in my first three months while in boot camp. With pure determination, strength, and conditioning, I believed that I would overcome and I could accomplish. Through all of the fatigue, I talked to myself and motivated myself to "just do it." Just "take the hill, Marine!" And so I worked hard to regain my strength by running, push-ups, running, sit-ups, more running and pull-ups—I ran and ran. I ran through all the pain, the heavy feet, and the fatigue. After three months of incredibly hard work, I finished the running portion of our unit's physical fitness test behind only one other Marine, Sam Anderson, who ran the required 3 miles barefoot for gosh sakes!

My Marine Corps career lasted a total of 10 years, and, other than a few minor incidents, I went, for the most part, symptom free. Now, after being diagnosed with multiple sclerosis (MS), I can reflect and recognize past symptoms and complications. While still on active duty, I began to notice my vision becoming blurred. Eyeglasses seemed to satisfy me for only six months when, in frustration, I returned to the eye doctor, who tweaked the prescription and sent me off with new glasses. At the time, no one thought about MS as the cause.

Mental fatigue would also come and go as I found myself experiencing periods of forgetfulness and hazy confusion. I became periodically confused and somewhat irritated; the mental fatigue made it difficult to follow conversations. Early one morning, Sgt. Mellons attempted to communicate instructions as we were about to begin the installation and start-up of new communications equipment. As if in a daze, I found it hard to understand and follow the instructions. I didn't get it! It was as if there was an invisible force field surrounding me that was preventing the flow of information. Physically present, while simply staring into space, I was mentally spent and unexplainably fatigued. Perhaps, I only needed some rest.

Shifting Gears

After 10 years of active military service, it was time to consider my future and my career options. Re-enlistment at this point would mean I was serious about making the military my career, and I would be eligible for retirement in 10 more years. Yet, there were no guarantees, since Congress was cutting military spending (career Marines), and I was having physical difficulties, now known to be early MS symptoms. We decided to shift gears, pack up our belongings, and go home to Wisconsin. There I began a successful career in manufacturing, first as a buyer (where I soon discovered I was on the wrong side of the desk), then as a sales professional specializing in CNC metalworking machinery. Finally, I decided to be an executive recruiter, a position in which I could continue to build on all my years of experience and knowledge while helping others grow in their careers.

The opportunity came by way of a nationally franchised executive recruiting business, which provided the safety net of "family" with superb training and support and access to some of the most technologically advanced services and systems. The world of recruiting is fun, it's complicated and challenging, and, it was the most rewarding thing I ever did—like an athlete who enjoys excelling in his chosen sport. The position meant that I would wear many different hats: career coach, business coach, sales, president, and business owner. With "my game head" on, I strategically juggled numerous projects and candidates while meeting the immediate needs of my clients. It was a comfortable fit.

My most memorable MS event (we all have them), was on a beautiful Saturday night at Miller Park in June of 2005. It was probably the largest crowd thus far for Miller Park, as Brewer fans filled the Stadium to watch rookie players Rickie Weeks, Prince Fielder, and J.J. Hardy in their first year of major league baseball. The Brewers were trailing Minnesota by one run when Fielder batted a solo homer. I remember the crowd leaping to their feet, the fireworks popping, and the stadium a buzz in cheers of excitement. Then the whole stadium began to spin.

Sitting down, attempting to "ride out" the now worsening dizzy feeling, left me thinking to myself "this is not good." It was as if I was observing the game from above, outside the stadium's open roof and from a distance. Everything before me seemed to spin. We didn't make it to the seventh inning stretch and famed Sausage Race. The long walk from the stadium to the car was evidence that something seriously wrong was happening to me. With wobbly legs, heavy feet, and everything appearing to move, I was carried fireman's style between two friends and tucked into the car.

As I visited with doctors and received referrals to many more doctors, I was often asked if I had ever experienced such symptoms in the past. Not thinking clearly, I reported "no" and that the symptoms just popped up out of nowhere. Now, after much personal research and education about my MS diagnosis, I can recall many earlier MS occurrences. Understanding MS explained certain misunderstood physical difficulties that I had encountered while serving on active duty in the United States Marine Corps. Yet, after all my MS research and visits with doctors, nothing had prepared me for the debilitating cognitive challenges that I would soon face.

Today's computer technology makes it easier than ever for an executive recruiter to stay organized and respond to a client's immediate needs. The scheduling of interviews, the important follow-ups, and the forwarding of detailed instructions can all be completed with a simple click of a mouse. While it was all right there, right in front of me on a computer screen, I was finding it harder and harder to understand the details. Even reading a resume was becoming frustrating. I would print it, look at it, recognize it as a resume, yet the words seemed to float as I stared at a piece of paper unable to understand it. As if I was attempting to navigate through a thick fog, the once routine tasks had somehow become confusing and difficult. Unknowingly, MS was interfering as this normally well-organized, detail-orientated executive recruiter was mentally fumbling.

In the office, sorting through numerous project details and planning my activities were becoming insurmountable as my energy weakened. Unknowingly, I began adapting by shortcutting my impeccable system of doing business. The hours of time spent gathering information from candidates was shortened as extreme mental fatigue was taking its toll on me. Secretly, I solicited the help of my administrative assistant, who was now charged with the responsibility of reviewing resumes and data and sorting the information based on client needs. Convincing myself that I could still do this, I maintained contact and provided clients with the now-shortcut details. Absentmindedness and difficulties communicating my thoughts made professional follow-up both difficult and embarrassing because I was attempting to adapt to something I did not know or understand. I was failing.

Early in my MS struggles, I pushed, kicked, and fought against the clear physical obstacles. Perhaps rolling backwards and losing ground, pushing and fighting even harder, I did the only thing I knew how to do—fight! Now, I was fighting for my life and my business and fighting to keep my head above water. Fighting as a Marine would know how, I would "take the hill!! Meanwhile, I naively accepted MS by convincing myself that MS was no problem. As an executive recruiter with MS, I can easily pull up to my desk in a wheelchair, be productive, and continue to grow my business while comfortably providing for my family. Just don't take away my ability to clearly and quickly think. I can work the business with my legs placed in a wheelchair, but just don't take my thoughts!

Now, with a smile, I reflect that my in-laws are two of the most adventurous and supportive individuals whom I have ever known, and Kathy is "loved" by them very much! We traveled the world, and, wherever the Marine Corps would take us, her parents were sure to come and visit. It was while traveling and sightseeing in the Blue Ridge Mountains when I first heard Judy (my mother-in-law) playfully announce that I needed to be careful because someday Kathy would push me off a cliff while I was seated in my wheelchair. We chuckled, got a good laugh, and I continued to hear the same "promise" several times over in our now 29 years of marriage.

Today, seated at my desk and contemplating my future with MS, that promise of being introduced to a wheelchair and a cliff is no longer funny. I find that my ability to think quickly "on my feet" has been impaired. This realization is the most painful part of my MS. Perhaps voice-recognition software will be of help on those days when my hands and fingers won't work right, but the forgetfulness is something new to me. My "on the fly" abilities to plan, strategize, and organize while navigating the many details with quick, complete, and professional follow through has been crippled. To be able to "think on my feet" was vital to my business success. I feared I had lost something. To what extent I did not know, but I knew something had changed, and I desperately needed help.

Tune Up

Yes, I had good days and bad days, but my cognitive difficulties seemed to increase throughout the day. I was struggling in my business activities and was beginning to have a slow, sinking feeling. Feeling desperate, needing help and immediate results, I was referred for a neuropsychological evaluation. I explained that I had been experiencing difficulty with my memory, concentration, and planning and that I seemed to become easily distracted. A neuropsychologist, Dr. Josie Matthais, listened with empathy as I described how difficult it had become to focus and how reading and understanding my own typed or handwritten notes was now a challenge to absorb.

As we chatted, I became more and more comfortable, perhaps feeling safe as Dr. Matthais understood when I communicated my difficulties following conversations, finding words, and losing my train of thought midsentence. An all-day battery of tests was performed to establish my current level of cognitive functioning. Tests measuring intellectual abilities, verbal comprehension skills, organizational skills, memory, and processing speed revealed difficulties on tasks that have increasing demand on processing speed and divided attention.

The result showed that my memory ranged from borderline low to average, and I seemed to perform poorly in the mornings. I was totally blown away with these findings about me and my MS. After a short break for lunch and some rest, came the challenging PASAT test. This is an auditory test requiring mental arithmetic of orally presented numbers, adding the first number of a sequence to the last number of the previous sequence. Perhaps challenging "fun" for most anyone, it was painfully frustrating for me. I had difficulties keeping up with the pace as I struggled, often teary eyed, while attempting to adapt and keep up with the test. I couldn't do it.

The important baseline had now been established, and, when I revisited Dr. Matthais one year later, I arrived uncharacteristically late. I had become lost while traveling roads that I had frequently traveled and with which I was expertly familiar. Frustrated and in urgent need of help, I explained how I thought that I was experiencing more cognitive loss. The retests confirmed my concern of mental decline in nearly all areas as I struggled to cope with the changes. My frustrations were limiting my life, and, with this realization and Dr. Matthais' help, I was able to begin a life-changing process of cognitive behavioral therapy.

The cognitive therapy began with my purchasing Dr. Burns' book, *Feeling Good*, and the daily logging of my feelings, thoughts, and situations. With all of the discipline and energy one might expect of a former Marine, I logged throughout the day and night. I wrote about daily frustrations on bad days and the associated stress or anger. I also wrote about the good days, having energy, and being productive. As I continued to log and later analyze for distorted thoughts, I wrote about my physical conditions and mental state, as well as my family and the apparent effects of my MS on them. It was very revealing as I learned how my thoughts were driving my feeling about myself and my situation. With continued therapy, I learned to view my world and life with MS in a more peaceful and accepting manner.

In business, I drove myself by setting annual goals and then broke those goals down into smaller monthly, weekly, and daily goals. In a military sense, my goals became marching orders, and I ordered myself with "have to" regular goals to be accomplished. My "should, have, and must" statements became expectations. They were demands that perhaps even those without MS would have difficulty achieving. With MS, that fighting would work against me, and I was unknowingly setting myself up for personal failure.

In just a few weeks, with continued logging, came the peaceful realization that I was no longer able to expertly perform the intense business practices while serving the immediate needs of my clients and candidates. This realization led to another and more important understanding. Although my family and friends would always be there for me and would understand and be supportive of me and my MS, my clients and candidates would not. After all, it's business, and they could not be expected to assume that role for me. Coming home from the office irritable, frustrated, and absolutely drained was not a good thing because I'm no good to my family and friends with my "brain housing group" being mush from pushing myself.

My life, my family, friends, and relationships are far more important, and, through continued logging and cognitive therapy, my thoughts, my attitude, and how I perceived my life and MS began to change. I started focusing on my strengths, my skills, and how I could continue to use them while protecting my true priorities. One lingering question remained: was I giving up and surrendering to MS or taking control and staying in the game?

Dousman Derby Days is our small town's annual carnival with kiddy rides, fireworks, and, of course, a beer tent complete with live music and dancing. The July event is like a high-school reunion as old friends and acquaintances become reunited and catch up on the latest news and events, with promises of "getting together sometime." Volunteers are needed in a food tent to help prepare and sell sandwiches for a local charitable organization, and I had volunteered. The line of hungry customers grew fast as the parade of fire engines, tractors, and marching bands was now over. I've been instructed to help out at the cash counter, where three dollars buys customers a big fat quarter-pound hot dog or a great-tasting bison sandwich with chips and a pickle.

With the cash box placed safely in front of me and the tent buzzing with noise and activity, I'm ready to take my first order. A lady pulls a 50 dollar bill from her purse and orders five sandwiches, and I fold. Without warning and in a very instant, my brain goes blank. I find myself somehow floating away as if my brain and body are not connected. Physically I am here inside this tent, while my head is out in space somewhere and unable to connect, unable to do simple math, and unable to make correct change.

Being lost in the moment can creep up at any time and any place and, like a scene from Star Trek with the transporter failing, my mind has suddenly "beamed" into outer space. During these times, my five senses (sight, hearing, taste, smell, and touch) are intact, yet it is difficult to comprehend and difficult to understand conversations. It is as if the words are there, I can hear them, and, for some reason, they are being blocked. It's troubling and it's frustrating and, as hard as I try for the moment, MS just will not allow my brain to work. The lady is waiting for her change.

Thankfully, there is plenty of help as I hand the 50 dollar bill to my friend Glenn and tell him—I can't. I leave the hot tent and stand in the coolness of a shade tree for a few moments and collect myself, observing the long lines at other booths. Dousman is a small town where everybody knows each other, and I have MS, so I adjust to my mental money jam and begin greeting the people in those long food lines. I can still help.

I am received by smiling faces with warm hugs and handshakes, friends and acquaintances inquire "how you doing" and tell me "I look well!" With cognitive challenges, "looks" aren't everything. "Doing great," I reply with positive affirmation, while suggesting this particular line has the best damn hot dogs and the bison sandwich is absolutely great! Oh, by the way, the line is shorter because the service is quicker!

We sell out of hot dogs in three hours, and, by 5:00 p.m., we have only enough bison sandwiches to feed five hungry volunteers. The opportunity to volunteer and stay in the game has left me full and satisfied.

Taking the Hill

While participating as a volunteer (handing out water) at the 2005 and 2006 MS 150 Best Dam Bike Tour, I made it a goal to get strong and participate as a rider in 2007—a huge challenge, since it was only a year ago that I was unable to ride up a small hill just 5 blocks from my home. Its 12:30 p.m. on Wednesday afternoon, and it's a typically hot and humid mid-July day, with only a couple of weeks left to train—and I'm riding! I've chosen this afternoon especially because of the particularly warm and humid weather to properly condition myself. To cover 75 miles each day, while allowing myself adequate rest stops, at an average speed of 14 mph, I will likely be pedaling in the warmer, perhaps more humid, part of the day.

I've only been riding for 15 miles, and the heat and humidity cause me to question my motivations. Is it unrealistic to expect the very best of myself, possibly setting goals so high that even those who do not have MS would have difficulty achieving? Perhaps I need to change my standards and expectations, understanding what's realistic and unrealistic? If only I could keep my head clear to think it through!" This weather is far different than it had been during my initial training.

It is January and, with the parking lot full, I think "damn," I'll have to park clear across the lot and walk. Being careful not to slip on the snow and ice, I am thinking about how crowded the "Y" is this morning and betting most people have begun their New Year's resolutions to a new lifestyle commitment of losing weight and getting in shape. I'm also wondering if I will get my favorite lane, the last lane, the one closest to the wall. It seems I need the comfort and security of the wall, should I tire while I swim.

This morning I'm already tired, both physically and mentally, and am too proud (embarrassed) to use the reserved disabled/handicap parking area. It seems at times like this, when I am foggy headed and feeling the all-over physical fatigue of heavy arms and legs, when I just want to lie down and rest—I become angry. Perhaps I just want to be left alone and not engage in conversation. It's too mentally tasking. I can feel the tightness of certain nerves and muscles in my head and frowning face, perhaps appearing angry. This is not me. Angry is not how I want to be perceived.

I have found the best time for my morning swim is between the hours of nine and 10 when the pool is conveniently roped for those adults who engage in water aerobics and for those who choose to swim laps. As I jump in, I find the water to be perfectly cool, perfectly cool because it is not breath taking. Perfectly cool because, as I swim, it keeps my body temperature cool, allowing me to "go the distance" before my body gives out from the "wet-noodle" effect of heat.

Today, I must share (my) lane with a female swimmer who seems to not mind my taking the wall side of the lane. Later I learned that she is a triathlete and has a friend with MS. As I swim, I pace myself with discipline to be sure that my competitive nature does not interfere with why I am here. In my past life, I may have had something to prove, a personal thing, as I would have secretly raced the person in the lane next to me. Now, conserving my energy, I pace myself and, with three full laps complete, I stop to rest because my arms and legs feel sluggish.

Observing other swimmers—they must be doing 20, 50, maybe even 100 laps—I push off and continue my swim. With four laps now complete, my swimming is reduced to lengths rather than laps as I rest at each end of the pool. My legs and arms seem heavier and harder to control, while my legs seem to drag and pedal under me. My arms have become harder to place out and ahead of me as it takes more effort to lift, place, and dig in the water. With another six lengths complete, I clumsily climb the ladder, grab the handles to steady myself, and shuffle to the bleachers, where I will sit and rest a few moments. Even with MS, I'm happy and grateful. It is progress, since not that long ago that I was unable to do one full lap!

In a bit of a haze and while concentrating on my balance, I sort of shuffle off to the locker room. What is interesting to me is that, as my workouts improve, the recovery time from mental and physical fatigue seems to improve. Although my shower, shave, and dressing may take a bit more time than fellow "Y" members and although I may still seem to shuffle out of the Y and to my car, the brief drive home or to the grocery store is all I need. My head is together and I seem to have nearly fully recovered the energy to grocery shop, run errands, or whatever! This is a marked improvement over my earlier days when swimming would have wiped me out for the entire day. Even when I felt a little worn out from going up the hill against MS, it was clear to me that I couldn't stop exercising. Riding for a cause would benefit others from these efforts, as long as I can hold my thoughts together.

It's a terrible thing, struggling daily with troubling questions about losing my mental edge. Whether mowing the lawn, swimming, or even while physically at rest watching Brewers baseball on TV, my mind is burdened with that haunting question: Will I keep my head together and maintain the bicycle on course for a safe ride? Finding an exercise routine that functions within the limits of my MS limits was crucial. The point was not to hold myself up to the standards of when I was on active duty as a Marine, but to take those fundamental skills and apply them as motivation to take the new hill. By remaining in motion, even on the hot and humid afternoon of the MS Bike Tour, I am not stopping and I will repeat it because, even though I may need assistance and proceed more deliberately, I am not stopping.

As I continued to ride through the draining humidity and heat, I was reminded of a story made famous by Dr. Charles Swindoll about a 19th century violinist named Nicolo Paganini. It seems Paganini was performing a difficult piece in front of a packed house when several strings broke on his violin, and Paganini, without missing a beat, not only was able to finish, but expertly performed an encore on the one remaining string. Charles Swindoll tells it best and relates this story to attitudes, with the reminder that we cannot change the inevitable. The only thing we can do is play on the one string we have, and that is our attitude.

"I am convinced that life is 10% what happens to me and 90% how I react to it. And so it is with you ... we are in charge of our attitudes," Swindoll concludes. This story remains pinned on a bulletin board above my desk, reminding me to be in charge of my attitudes, daily. With my cognitive therapy, I now recognize such situations and can manually maneuver by logging and getting back in control of my thoughts and emotions. I may have been slowed and weakened a bit from a slight lapse, but soon, like riding a bike, I'm pedaling, in motion, and moving forward again.

Suddenly, I'm awakened from this slight lapse of attention as I find myself struggling to maintain control of my bicycle. I am steering, with my arms locked straight, but the soft, loose gravel of the roadside shoulder has sucked me in. A friend and experienced biker told me that I should stop and manually maneuver the bike back onto the paved road should I ever find myself in such a situation. Good advice! The shoulder had acted like a vacuum sucking the narrow tires deep into the loose gravel. It was everything I could do to come to a controlled stop.

So it is with MS, my attitudes, and my emotions for dealing with the physical and cognitive slowdowns. If the uncontrolled feelings remain in motion, then they tend to suck me into the emotional gravel, leading to a crash. When my feelings toward MS are understood and I can pause and pace myself through the dragging moments, then I can return to motion without damage to myself or others. It is a successful method to a functional path.

With the cognitive and physical difficulties of MS on board with me for the ride, it seems like a good opportunity to chart and think through my best path for the MS150 Best Dam Bike Tour. In our first year, we have 33 team members assembled at the starting line of the MS150 Best Dam Bike Tour. Proudly, our riders don their "Team Copaxone" bike jerseys like military uniforms and ride off as a unit. For now, we truly feel like we are a part of something, something big, a team, "Peppy Pedalers" and "Team Copaxone." The fresh air, peacefulness, and exercise help me to "clear my head and think."

With one day down and only 50 more miles to go, I have decided to break away from my group and draft faster riders because I want to be at the finish line at about 1:30 p.m. Last year, a group of us with MS began greeting riders and autographing their placards, which proved to be a very emotionally moving experience. Unbelievable, as riders of all ages, who had just ridden 150 miles to help our Wisconsin chapter raise more than $1.6 million dollars for continued research, broke down in tears as people with MS with canes, wheelchairs, or scooters were greeting them, hugging them, thanking them for their support, and autographing their MS150 numbers placard.

Although inexperienced at drafting, I find it helps "pull" me along at faster speeds and with less effort on my part. Like getting into a groove or riding a wave, I need only to maintain balance and motion and stay with the pack. It can be dangerous when I cannot see what obstacles lie ahead, since my vision is obscured by the rider immediately in front of me. Yet, I'm on a mission to complete the ride and be at the finish line by 1:30 p.m., so I have faith and trust in those riders ahead of me—much the same way we trust in those who have ridden life with MS before us. We have learned from them, from our doctors, and from the extensive research that exists on the subject of living with MS. We need now only maintain balance and avoid those "potholes" and other obstacles that may lie ahead. Here, there is no dumping—only mutual support.

More hills! The heat, humidity, and hills are beginning to take their toll on me. I'm weakening, pedaling at a much slower 9-mph clip, and I'm struggling to maintain my balance as a brother and sister approach me from behind. We introduce ourselves and chat along the route for the next seven or so miles. The couple appears to be in their mid to upper forties and wear matching MS150 jerseys, and, because I'm wearing a "yes, I have MS" pin on my back, they take notice and comment with encouraging words. Their younger brother, who has MS, walks only with the assistance of a cane and often uses a scooter. We share a goal.

At this point, having someone to chat with is a great help to me as I find myself focusing on more than my current status and struggles to maintain posture and balance. They understand the physical symptoms of MS, and now they are learning all about the cognitive effects and the associated daily challenges. They learn how, much like riding a bike, I have learned to live with MS by remaining physically active and mentally challenged, balancing my day and my life. It is a slower and modified workout, but it helps me to get to the end. It is a winning MS ride.

Popping the Clutch

Living with MS is about maintaining balance while making choices, setting priorities, staying focused, and moving forward. In the beginning, I only knew that I needed help and, as if driving that old Ford dump truck, I circled and circled, trying new things, new doctors, new diets, and supplements, and all the while "searching for the right hill."

My commitment set the stage for distorted thoughts and, thus, unrealistic expectations, ultimately leading to embarrassing letdowns, missed deadlines, and unfulfilled promises. Painfully, I had shut down the business and applied for Social Security, thus closing that chapter of my life and for all the right reasons. I concluded that clients and candidates trusted and depended on me to professionally fulfill their immediate needs—something I could no longer do.

Intense and running low on fuel, I parked and put on the brakes in time to find Dr. Matthais. The "movie" in this case became a learning and life-changing process. Logging my feelings, situation, and thoughts every morning, afternoon, and night, I learned to drive past my defeating and distorted thoughts, "parking" on the right "hill" and ready to keep moving. The transferring of business records, data, and activities to our Milwaukee affiliates was the practical, professional, and correct action. With the transfer complete and official notifications sent out, my priorities were in clear focus and my future was opened. Mentally relaxed and at peace, I began to contemplate the often-heard business theory that "time is money."

We can spend our time on productive projects or seemingly waste it in unproductive projects or interests. With MS, I find myself daily evaluating how and where I spend my time—more importantly, how and where I spend my very valuable and limited energy and who I spend it with. Energy comes in two facets, one being physical and the other mental. Sometimes, while I am physically at rest, my mind may still be active, thereby allowing me to continue in my writing, planning, and organizing activities. At other times, my mind needs rest, and, during these times, all activity requiring mental thought or energy is put on hold. Although I might enjoy certain physical activity, I am generally alone or with trusted (safe) people.

Mental energy can be consumed during focused, organized, and productive activity. Energy can also be spent during valuable social activities with family and friends. Being there, both mentally and physically, is extremely important. Whether at play, during leisure time, or in serious discussions, I treat energy as a valuable resource to be protected and conserved for my family and friends. Time and energy may also be drained from me by being around negative people or activities. They seemingly come around in need of an emotional boost and take something valuable from me. Some people just want to "dump," perhaps complaining about work, associates, money, or lack of money. What is certain for me is that when they dump their negativity, they are now feeling better, leaving me drained of important energy.

Safe people understand and respect my need to rest and recharge. They include my family and close friends, and they understand my need for quiet time and the momentary mental lapses. They understand my MS and how morning time is for me, my exercises and my productive activities. This may seem a bit selfish, but some people cannot or will not understand or respect me and my needs, while sucking out valuable energy. With my limited physical and cognitive resources, who is more self-serving?

My MS is progressive. As each disabling wave hits, I'm down for a week or more, followed by another week or two of recovery, requiring frequent and regular rest. There are some good days and then, for no apparent reason, I get hit by another wave. It is a vicious MS cycle, slowly getting worse as the waves keep washing in and I start all over again. My priorities are my health and exercise and my relationships with family and friends. If I slow the progression of MS lesions, then perhaps I can slow the intervals and the severity of the waves. Maybe I will shorten the down time and perhaps even require less recovery time. All this could lead to more, and certainly valuable, "good days" for my benefit and the benefit of my family and friends.

Swimming, biking, and yoga are my exercises of choice. Whether I "feel" like it or not, whether I am up to it or not, I exercise. Personally, I am absolutely convinced of the physical and mental benefits because I seemingly have more energy and am more cognitively "with it." I also stay involved, and thus in mental motion, as a volunteer Peer Supporter with the Wisconsin Chapter of the National MS Society, as well as a member of the Advocacy and Government Affairs Committee. Through presenting "MS and Career Crossroads" workshops, my executive-recruiting experience may help those with MS contemplating their future and career changes.

That's the balance I have searched for and have found through exercise, by staying involved, and by staying "in motion" because one seems to impact and drive the other. By doing so, I have been able to constructively work through an otherwise emotionally draining and painful process. Knowing my MS cognitive limitations, while pacing and balancing my energy and mental stamina, will be an ongoing learning process. Although I may "look good," I can confidently exclaim that I didn't give up and I didn't quit. I have simply learned where to come to a rest and how to "pop the clutch," get started again, and open a new chapter in my life.

Reflecting upon my 10 years of intense active duty, I am now seated next to Kathy in the reviewing booth overlooking the parade deck at MCRD San Diego. Thirty-one years ago, I stood on this very same parade deck and received my Eagle, Globe, and Anchor. The platoons, all marching in unison, are taking their positions while the Marine Band plays on. With a height of six-foot four, our son, Kyle, is easily spotted. He appears to be struggling with his attempts to hold back the tears. I understand, as I am doing my best to choke back my own tears.

The graduation ceremony is brilliant and true to Marine tradition, with all of the expected pageantry, precision, honor, and pride. Kyle will never forget his 12 weeks of boot camp training, his drill instructors, and this fateful graduation day. No longer able to hold back, my tears flow as the band begins playing the Marine Corps Hymn, and Kyle smiles, not much, but I catch it. It is a familiar smile, one that comes from deep down and in the heart. It's something only a Marine understands. No matter where he is or what he is doing, from now and forever, when hearing the Marine Corps Hymn, Kyle will stand tall and proud, as those before him have done, and will remember who and what he is—a United States Marine.

With a deep, throaty voice, the drill instructor pronounces Platoon 1005—dismissed! I stand with my cane in hand and navigate the stairs, wary of all the eager parents flooding the parade deck to greet their new Marine. At this moment, MS is a distant concern, and I realize that a great life is in front of Kyle and remains inside me. Hugging Kyle is like hugging a tree. Solid! I remember standing tall and being in that state of top physical condition, military lean, built, and confident. It is a sort of cocky confidence, as if saying—charge, full speed ahead! It is all about standing together as Marines and now so much more. It was for different reasons, but, perhaps, we are proud of each other.

As for this retired Marine, parked on the hill, I'm ready to take on any and all challenges, including those invisible MS cognitive hurdles ... Oooh Rah!

Mental Sharpening Stones and Perspectives

1. Whatever your discipline level when your MS was diagnosed, rediscover it and engage it to remain active.
2. Where appropriate, seek and welcome MS-trained counseling to support focusing your energies and maximizing your strengths.
3. Seek out safe people, close family and friends, those who do not drain energy from you by dumping their personal problems into your life.
4. When experiencing cognitive challenges, allow your mind to rest and regain mental energy.
5. Remember that we cannot change the inevitable, only our attitude and our perceptions.

CHAPTER 5

Psychological Coping: Interchanging Puzzle Pieces to Form a Whole

Sharon S. Fedderly, PhD

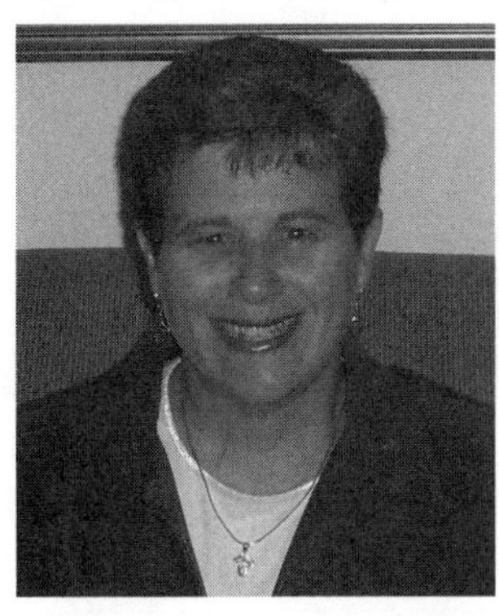

Dr. Sharon Fedderly is a clinical psychologist with Health Psychology Associates, a private-practice group in Milwaukee, Wisconsin. From both her prior experience as a staff psychologist on a rehabilitation medicine unit of the University of Wisconsin Hospital in Madison and her current clinical work, Dr. Fedderly has worked with patients with multiple sclerosis, from their early diagnosis to later treatment.

I developed my love of jigsaw puzzles as a young child. All shapes, all sizes, all patterns—I enjoyed them all. And as I grew older, the more challenging the puzzles were, the more I loved putting them together. Family and friends were aware of my interest and emerging skill and often bought me puzzles for birthdays, holidays, other special occasions. By the age of 10 or 11, I had a sizeable collection.

It was at that same age that I made an interesting discovery. I noticed that several of the puzzles manufactured by a particular company were the same size and also had the same cuts. That is, the shapes of the pieces and their interlocking patterns were the same in several of my puzzles. Only the picture patterns on the pieces were different. Quickly, I put together three of these puzzles, placed them side by side, and called my parents into my bedroom. I then took a piece from one puzzle and switched it with a piece from the second puzzle, and then swapped pieces between the second and third. Immediately, they were able to see how the pieces were indeed interchangeable. This later prompted my mother to take me into the hobby shop where the puzzles had been purchased and share my discovery with the owner. Although the owner was not entirely pleased with what I was showing him, I never realized until recently how that discovery would have relevance to my work as a clinical psychologist in private practice.

My exposure to multiple sclerosis (MS) has come from both family and friends who have the disease and my clinical work. These experiences, in combination with my work with patients with chronic conditions impacting their cognitive functioning (medical, psychiatric, or both), provide information that can be useful to the MS community. In this chapter, therefore, I take my "pieces" of experience with clinically diverse populations and, like I did with the jigsaw puzzle example, apply them to the cognitive challenges of MS.

Shifting Gears

Being diagnosed with a chronic and often progressive condition sets in motion a number of profound changes in how one views oneself, one's purpose, and one's activities. A person may ask, "Who am I, now that I have this disease?" If a person's definition of himself is based primarily on his profession, hobbies, or other activities and those pursuits are or may be compromised by the disease, self-esteem can suffer and an identity crisis can ensue. Think, for example, of the professional baseball player who loses the use of his pitching arm, or the artist who loses her sight.

As the questions emerge about a person's changed sense of self, other changes are simultaneously occurring in that person's family system and larger social context. Family roles may change in terms of who is the primary breadwinner, who handles the parenting responsibilities, who manages the finances, and so on. A person may experience shifts or losses in her social support network. Some friends and colleagues will "step up"; others will be less able or willing to do so. This latter scenario may be due to others' discomfort with the change in the person they once knew. Friends and colleagues may also become more distant out of the fear of not knowing the right way to respond.

It then becomes necessary and very important for individuals with a chronic condition like MS to articulate how they want to be treated by others. This can be a daunting task for people who have newly diagnosed MS and may not yet know what they need and want from others.

The experience of these changes and losses marks the beginning of a grieving process. People grieve the loss of the way they previously lived their life. They also grieve the loss of the dream of how they expected their life to be in the future. A person may go through phases of grief not unlike those described in the death and dying literature, such as denial, protest, or despair.[1] For some, the process may be time-limited; for others, it may come in waves, manifesting itself during one phase of life, then lying dormant until they face a new challenge or a new loss.

Over time, and under the right conditions, a person with a chronic or progressive condition stops being victimized and controlled by their illness. A degree of adaptation takes place such that symptoms and limitations are taken into consideration, but they do not hold the individual hostage as they might have in the earlier stages. *The individual makes peace with the enemy.* A person takes the approach, "I have this disease, which challenges who I am and what I do, but I also have ways of keeping the disease in check and tempering its impact."

Looking specifically at a person with MS, this could mean using a mobility device to prevent a fall, rather than repeatedly experiencing falls, as well as the fear, anger, and frustration that may accompany the falls. It could also mean making *cognitive* accommodations. A person may develop strategies that minimize the effects of delayed or disrupted thinking, distorted visual perceptions, and memory lapses.

It is important to emphasize that the process of adaptation is never linear. I believe this is so even when one experiences a single, nonprogressive change in one's functioning or experience. For example, even when a child experiences the divorce of his or her parents at age 10, a degree of adaptation must take place as that child grows into adulthood and confronts new challenges related to that earlier event. Who will be present at graduations, weddings, and other lifecycle events? How will step-parents be integrated or excluded? The adaptation to a condition like MS can be even more complex, inasmuch as the disease is characterized by symptoms that can emerge and then go underground in an unpredictable manner.

Challenges and setbacks are to be expected. A man who prides himself in taking care of the family finances may find it necessary to share the task with spouse when thinking skills become disrupted. The acknowledgement of this change prompts a new phase of grieving. The sharing of the task is an example of a new type of adaptation to the disease.

For some individuals, an exacerbation of MS symptoms necessitates a change in schedule, responsibilities, or even career. Nevertheless, this process does not have to lead to permanent despair; it has the potential to be empowering, providing the individual with an opportunity to develop a new sense of mastery. How a person makes the shift from grieving to adaptation and empowerment very much depends on a number of important factors: (1) the ability to identify and play to one's strengths; (2) the removal of obstacles; (3) the ability to pace oneself; (4) the ability to set limits; (5) the successful search for meaning in one's life; (6) the use of supportive others; and (7) the ability to be flexible, open, and make use of humor.

Strategy #1: Identifying and Playing to One's Strengths

The concept of capitalizing on one's innate assets or learned skills is one that makes sense to everyone: a person who knows how to present ideas in a logical, interesting, and easy-to-understand way may be one who is suited to a profession such as teaching, writing, or law. Conversely, a person who cannot hold a tune should probably shy away from a career as a vocalist. Under optimal circumstances of physical, cognitive, and emotional health, we all come into the world with different strengths and talents, as well as limitations. Our goal in life is not to try to make ourselves strong in all areas, but to pursue a path (socially, intellectually, and professionally) that draws upon those strengths and minimizes the impact of the limitations.

We probably all know people who honed their talents, pursued realistic dreams based on those talents, and ultimately succeeded in realizing those dreams. We can probably also identify people who are masters of self-sabotage: they repeatedly "shoot themselves in the foot" and do not possess the insight or the motivation to modify their behaviors to create positive outcomes for themselves.

This strategy is particularly important in the context of the cognitive symptoms of MS. Playing to a one's strengths may take the form of focusing one's energies on those pursuits that are unaffected by those symptoms, or being selective about one's activities to minimize the potential triggering of cognitive symptoms. A person who can no longer process information as quickly would therefore avoid those employment or volunteer opportunities in which information is presented at a rapid-fire pace and must be processed and responded to quickly. Another individual who has learned that his word-finding problems increase the more fatigued he becomes would want to refrain from activities requiring prolonged physical or intellectual exertion.

※ Strategy #2: Removing the Obstacles

Another way to minimize the impact of cognitive symptoms and allow a person to live a strong and productive life involves the use of accommodations. Accommodations can take a number of forms, such as the daily planner filled with important information to remember plus a to-do list, the use of auto-pay services for bills, the setting up of a work environment with fewer distractions, or the taking of an antidepressant to counter the mood effects of MS that also undermine cognitive skills. Such strategies can be viewed as removing the obstacles to accessing one's strengths.

Sarah is a corporate executive in her 40s who was diagnosed with MS approximately 15 years ago. Although her initial symptoms were more physical, cognitive symptoms developed several years later, including slower information processing, word-finding problems, a decreased ability to focus, memory difficulties, and impaired decision-making and organizational skills.

Currently, Sarah's symptoms vary in their severity. During an exacerbation, they worsen. At other times, they are either less noticeable or easier to manage.

Sarah has come to learn about and cope with her cognitive symptoms in a number of significant ways. Playing to her strengths, she has selected the type of employment situation that capitalizes on her analytical skills and other areas of expertise, but that is less cognitively demanding than the types of positions she sought prior to her diagnosis. For Sarah, this has meant a move from a larger, high-pressure corporation to one that is smaller and less stressful.

Sarah structures her work environment to maximize her focus, and she uses a number of mnemonic strategies and memory aids to minimize the impact of her memory diffi-

culties. For example, she asks an assistant to take notes during business meetings in which the exchange of information is likely to be quick and from multiple sources simultaneously. In addition, when Sarah is having a bad day with her physical or cognitive symptoms, she works from home.

Sarah conserves her professional energy by simplifying other aspects of her life: She uses the auto-pay function for most of her bills; she is selective in her social and volunteer activities; and she seeks out assistance and support from others—whether they are her family, her neighbors, or her spiritual community. Most importantly, Sarah has learned to become very attuned to her symptoms and takes preventive and corrective action to protect and maintain her cognitive abilities and overall level of functioning. She consults with her neurologist and internist during an exacerbation and seeks out new strategies in the face of new cognitive and physical challenges.

In addition to making use of accommodations there can also be benefits to aggressively "taking on" cognitive symptoms and fighting their possible progression. Sudoku, crossword puzzles, and reading, as well as physical exercise, have been found to be beneficial in keeping cognitive skills sharp. A recent series of studies has shown a relationship between exercise therapy and increased muscle strength and mobility in people with MS.[2] Further research is needed to understand the neurologic mechanisms by which exercise—both physical and cognitive—can slow the progression of the disease.

To conclude, playing to a person's strengths in the face of cognitive MS symptoms may involve a delicate balance of working around the symptoms, avoiding excessive cognitive and physical exertion, and simultaneously keeping the brain and body stimulated.

1. Pursue employment and other activities that involve cognitive skills unaffected by MS.
2. Avoid excessive physical or intellectual activity that could create fatigue and prompt or exacerbate cognitive symptoms.
3. Engage in regular mental and physical exercise to keep skills sharp. Consult with a physical therapist for exercise guidelines that are appropriate for you.
4. Consider consulting with an occupational therapist, who can assist you in structuring your work and home environments in a way that allows you to access your strengths.
5. Make use of organizational strategies, memory aids and techniques, and computerized services that minimize the impact of cognitive difficulties.

Strategy #3: Setting Limits

When faced with a chronic condition like MS, one has to ask the questions, "Where do my strengths lie now?" and "What do I need to put in place now so I can experience success?" A person who was able at one time to simultaneously juggle several responsibilities might now approach responsibilities one at a time, as well as choose those responsibilities that are manageable. Decisions may need to be made on a regular basis as to what task takes priority: engaging in an activity involving mental effort or pursuing a physically oriented task. Rather than fall prey to a victim mentality of "I can't do this anymore" or "I am helpless," the focus shifts to "here is what I *can* do," "this is what I *can* manage," and "here is what I have to offer *now*."

In the 1970s and 80s, books about assertiveness exploded on the pop psychology scene. Titles like *Don't Say Yes When You Want to Say No*[3] and *When I Say No I Feel Guilty*[4] were big sellers, and many workshops and therapists made assertiveness training their focus. The purpose of these books was to assist people in advocating for themselves and setting limits with others.

Many of us struggle with taking on tasks, problems, and responsibilities that we should probably defer to someone else. We feel the need to do it all. Sometimes we pay the price for overdoing it, whether it is increased anxiety, stress-related physical symptoms such as headaches and gastrointestinal disorders, or strained relationships with those who love us and feel worried about all we are taking on.

The unequivocal battle cry for those with chronic health conditions needs to be "When I Set Limits, I Stay Healthy." This echoes a verse from the Jewish text *Ethics of the Fathers*, which states, "If I am not for myself, who will be for me? And if I am only for myself, what am I? And if not now, when?"[5] The bottom-line message is not about selfishness but, rather, *self-protection*. In fact, there is a savings in taking time to relax because, in the long run, "recharging our batteries" allows us to be more available to others, more engaged in our activities, and more productive.

The words, "I'm sorry, I can't" can be hard to say, yet the cost of not saying them is one that cannot be afforded. People with a psychiatric condition such as schizophrenia or bipolar disorder may not be able to work full-time or take on too many stressful responsibilities, lest they experience an acute psychotic episode or a manic or depressed state. Extreme levels of stress and muscle tension can take their toll on *anyone's* cognitive functioning. A state of being overwhelmed can lead to impaired decision-making, memory difficulties, and disorganization.

Where cognitive compromise is already a concern, adding unnecessary stress to the mix is truly adding insult to injury. Denial of this fact can be dangerous. Although exacerbations of MS symptoms may be a reality of the disease, protecting one's mental health by setting reasonable limits can have preventive value in terms of the onset, severity, and long-term impact of an exacerbation.[6]

How to Set Limits

1. Be selective about what responsibilities you are willing and able to take on.
2. Learn to say "no" without feeling selfish or guilty.
3. Avoid unnecessary stress when possible.

Strategy #4: Pacing

Pacing oneself is a companion process to limit-setting. Unfortunately, it is challenging enough to say "no" to people, opportunities, additional activities, and responsibilities. Pacing oneself in our society takes the word "challenge" to an exponentially higher level. That is because pacing runs counter to the current state of our world.

We have come to expect that, with a click of a computer key, we can communicate instantly with someone on the other side of the world. Unfortunately, this amazing ability can lead us to set unrealistic time demands on ourselves. It is as if we have to keep up with technology: the world is moving at high speed, so we need to do the same. We live in a world where things have to be done yesterday, where "Type A" behavior is rewarded, and where "multitasking"—a word that did not exist before this century—is expected if not demanded.

Yet pacing is critical to the management of a chronic condition. During my work a number of years ago in a pain management program, pacing was emphasized again and again as essential to effective pain management. The act of "overdoing it," which is driven by guilt, frustration, or external pressure, can create disequilibrium—a state in which body, mind, and emotions seem out of balance—that can set a person back for days, weeks, months, or more. Pacing requires recognizing and heeding one's body signals.

Think of the "maximum load" or "maximum capacity" signs posted on elevators, busses, and airplanes. Add a few more pounds beyond that maximum load and risk a malfunction, worse yet, a crash. The same could be said when the body is taxed beyond its capacity. The body may start to ache, the brain may "shut down" and be less efficient in processing information, and a person may experience a variety of negative emotions, from frustration to anger to worry and despair.

Now, think of an individual with MS. If such an individual experiences greater cognitive confusion, word-finding problems, or an impaired ability to make decisions toward the end of a day, it makes sense to program in "recharging" breaks throughout the day that could prevent the onset of those cognitive symptoms. *A daily nap can make the difference in cognitive sharpness for a number of people with MS.* For others, two 15-minute "power naps" in a chair are more beneficial than lying down for an hour.

People with MS must do a continuous cost-benefit analysis, asking whether short-term results are better than longer-term productivity and maintenance of functioning. Although the idea of running one more errand, taking care of one more work responsibility, or scheduling one extra meeting can be very compelling, it can also be fuel to the MS symptom fire. It is imperative to given oneself permission to take it slower and take it easy.

Marie is a 45-year-old who was diagnosed with MS in her late 20s. Like Sarah, her cognitive symptoms emerged later and included short-term memory difficulties, slowed mental processing, and frequent instances of losing things, like her keys or glasses. When she became a mother and continued to experience significant exacerbations, Marie found that she could no longer juggle the demands of parenting with her work as a paralegal.

Since that time, Marie has created a lifestyle and daily routine that is protective of her cognitive, physical, and emotional functioning. For example, Marie is uncompromising about taking a daily nap and feels strongly that getting ade-

quate sleep is key to minimizing the impact of her condition on her life. A woman known for being exceptionally warm and caring, Marie has learned to say "no" to others and sometimes has to cancel commitments in the interest of conserving her resources and containing her symptoms.

Marie volunteers at her local MS Society chapter, speaking with individuals with newly diagnosed MS and assisting with fundraising. She volunteers at her daughter's school and does proofreading for her family. The latter plays to her strength as a lover of the English language and literature.

Marie plans to enter into a business venture with another family member, but she recognizes that she will have to consider the state of her condition as the business plan moves forward. For example, Marie is aware that she will need to program breaks into her day and may need to curtail her involvement and delegate responsibilities to others during exacerbations. In order to add this responsibility to her life, Marie realizes that she must also subtract out other responsibilities.

How to Pace Yourself

1. Program in "guilt-free" breaks, naps, quiet time, etc. to prevent fatigue that could undermine cognitive functioning.
2. Resist the temptation to overdo or set unrealistic deadlines.
3. Avoid "multitasking" whenever possible.

Strategy #5: Searching for Meaning

According to psychiatrist Viktor Frankl, a person's search for meaning is his "primary motivational force." A survivor of the Auschwitz concentration camp during World War II, he describes how a manuscript he had written that was ready for publication had been confiscated by the Nazis. He states that his desire to rewrite that manuscript helped him survive the trials of his confinement and writes, "I am sure that this reconstruction of my lost manuscript in the dark barracks of a Bavarian concentration camp assisted me in overcoming the danger of collapse."[7]

Frankl believed that we can discover meaning in life in three possible ways: by doing a deed, by experiencing a value (such as love, nature, or culture), and by suffering. But how does one transform a memory lapse, a sudden inability to recognize a loved one, or an inability to organize one's thoughts into something meaningful? This is not going to be an instantaneous shift. Again, one moves from grieving to adaptation. Reframing a negative change in cognitive functioning into a positive opportunity can only occur once the loss—of functioning, control, or both—is acknowledged, processed, and integrated into one's sense of self. This is a core feature of psychotherapeutic work with trauma clients.[8]

Once a person has moved from grief to adaptation, the search for meaning may take the form of sharing those experiences with others who know those symptoms but, up until that moment, never quite understood them, talked about them, or knew what they could do about them. It could also involve advocacy at the individual, community, or larger political level. Some find meaning in the religious or spiritual realm. Others report that they find meaning in reprioritizing their lives to make family, rather than professional success, primary.

Joanna is a college professor who lost her 4-year-old son in an automobile accident in which Joanna was driving. Her car was broadsided by another vehicle. Joanna was, herself, badly injured in the accident but was conscious enough at the time of the crash to see that her son was dead. This traumatic event resulted in Joanna experiencing posttraumatic stress disorder, a psychiatric condition characterized by a persistent re-experiencing of the traumatic event in the form of flashbacks, dreams, or disruptive thoughts. Other symptoms of this disorder include avoidance of anything associated with the traumatic event, as well as a significant level of emotional distress that interferes with sleep, concentration, and mood.[9]

Once Joanna recovered physically from the accident and went back to her professional and other responsibilities, she found herself struggling, both emotionally and cognitively. Staying focused in the classroom was difficult, as were previously simple tasks such as recording and organizing her students' grades. Joanna found herself easily "triggered" by thoughts, images, and emotions associated with the accident. She avoided the intersection where the accident occurred, as well as situations involving young children. Flashbacks of the accident would occur frequently while Joanna was driving, causing her to have to pull off the road, reorient, and calm herself down before proceeding again. Joanna forgot appointments, had to cancel classes, and had difficulty keeping track of her finances. Her relationships suffered.

Joanna's road to healing began through a combination of activities, including her participation in a grief support group for parents who had lost a child, her involvement in psychotherapy, and her increased availability to her students, supporting them in their own personal struggles. She established a fund in her son's memory at a local hospital and volunteered there. She restructured her courses and began to teach subject material that allowed her to channel her feelings of loss into creative energy. Joanna found comfort and inspiration from the Native American culture and incorporated the concept of "connectedness" into her work. She published a book of poetry about her grief experience. Over time, Joanna became recognized as a community resource for grieving parents and established an annual memorial service at her university.

Joanna sought out a neuropsychological evaluation of her cognitive skills, which confirmed the negative impact of her emotional trauma on her intellectual functioning. She benefited from the recommendations provided by this evaluation and made some significant changes in the way she approached the logistics of teaching and grading. She used strategies that minimized her memory and organizational challenges, while setting limits with colleagues and being more selective about her commitments.

It has now been more than 12 years since the accident and loss of her son, and the healing process is active and ongoing. Joanna has to commit herself to finding meaning in her life on a regular basis and admits that this is not always easy. At the same time, Joanna believes that there are aspects of her traumatic loss that have been a gift to her, albeit bittersweet. Her tragic experience has helped her to discover previously untapped strengths within her, as well as to feel a deeper empathy for others.

Joanna's story demonstrates that cognitive challenges—resulting from posttraumatic stress, MS, or any other condition—do not preclude a person from accessing other internal strengths, developing new skills, and participating in activities that are meaningful and fulfilling.

Successfully Searching for Your Own Meaning

1. Seek out those experiences that move you toward the future (for example, something with a worthwhile and attainable goal) and make you feel good about yourself.
2. Consider pursuing attainable "I've always wanted to do this" activities that have been put indefinitely on hold. Weigh the costs and benefits, and if it is possible, "just do it."
3. Try to engage in activities that transform your limitations and challenges into something positive that benefits others, as well as yourself. Ask yourself, "How can I make a difference in other people's lives or in the world?"

Strategy #6: Recognizing the Importance of Others

Many studies in the mental-health literature underscore the importance of social support as a "stress buffer."[10,11] People with clinical depression benefit from social interactions with positive, supportive others, despite their desire in many cases to socially withdraw. Alcoholics Anonymous and other similar programs draw heavily on the power of social support to assist people in the addiction recovery process. None of us functions in a vacuum, and most of us function best in some kind of social context. Other people can also be critically important if one has chronic health issues.

Even if a person's social environment is relatively small, or if a person is socially isolated, there are a number of ways of accessing greater social support. It can be through support groups (MS Society chapters offer such groups regularly), volunteer work, or religious or other spiritual institutions or through joining groups centered around a common hobby, craft, or other area of interest.

In conditions affecting cognitive functioning, the other person can be an auxiliary brain, a partner in helping one set limits and pace, a partner in helping one find meaning, or one who supports and facilitates a person's use of their strengths. In short, they can be stress buffers and/or energy conservers. At times, and in limited doses, others can also function as co-mourners or a shoulder when the grieving process intensifies.

John, a 50-year-old factory worker with a love of hunting and other wilderness activities, suffered a massive heart attack and required emergency bypass surgery. Twenty-four hours after the surgery, John had a stroke that resulted in right-sided weakness and permanent short-term memory difficulties. John was unable to remember events that had occurred during his day and often repeated himself, unaware of what he had said previously. John also had difficulty remembering the steps to different skills he had long mastered, such as making arrows and bow strings for hunting. His right-sided weakness made it difficult for him to shoot a bow, canoe, or participate in tasks requiring physical labor. Books were frustrating because he could not retain what he had read. Television shows with story lines were impossible for him to follow. All of this was a source of great distress to John.

With the steadfast help of his wife, Cindy, John was able to rebuild his life. Cindy, who also loves the outdoors, made sure that John participated in hunting trips. She educated his friends about short-term memory loss so they could provide the right amount of support and supervision that kept John safe but involved. Cindy encouraged John to contact friends who also made arrows and bow strings to come to their home, show John how to make them again, and have him write down the steps. She structured their home environment to make it easier for John to find various things around the house. She cued him to use his memory aids, such as notebooks and reminders posted in prominent places, but always treated him lovingly, respectfully, and patiently, never criticizing his repetitive questions or comments.

Over time, John has been able to relearn the crafts and skills he had lost. With some improvement in his right-sided function, he has resumed bow hunting, using a bow adapted to his level of strength. John and Cindy continue to participate in a variety of wilderness activities. They watch educational television because the single theme of the programs is easier for John to understand. In addition, John is a volunteer at both his local community center and an archery shop, where he connects with others who share his passion for bow hunting and the outdoors.

For the person experiencing the cognitive symptoms of MS, the other person may be the assistant at work who takes notes during meetings to make sure the critical points are remembered. Or the other can be the family member who removes distractions and simplifies family tasks to maximize focus and minimize fatigue. Finally, the other person can just be the friends and colleagues who reaffirm the person's importance in their lives.

Steve, age 55, is an engineer who was diagnosed with MS during his twenties. A man with chronic and progressive symptoms, Steve has come to be physically dependent on his wife, Ann, and on attendant care. Ironically, during his early professional life, Steve was instrumental in developing the prototype for the wheelchair that he now uses.

Cognitive symptoms have accompanied Steve's physical challenges, including memory lapses, decreased attention span, and difficulties with visual perception. As his MS has progressed, Steve has focused his efforts on reaching out to others: family, friends, and other people with MS. No longer able to work as an engineer, he has found a position with a medical equipment company, conducting telephone surveys about customer satisfaction.

Connecting with others is critical to his coping. Steve sometimes defers to Ann when faced with tasks requiring more-complex thinking skills (for example, long sequences of steps, tasks requiring sustained attention). Ann is his confidant, his primary source of cognitive and emotional support, and his number one fan.

Others, therefore, can play a powerful role in the adjustment to and management of cognitive MS symptoms. Sarah, as noted above, relies on her assistant for tasks requiring attention and memory. She also looks to family, neighbors, and her community for assistance and applies the concept of "it takes a village"[12] to individuals with MS. Both Sarah and Marie find fulfillment in "giving back" when they can, either at the individual level or by their volunteer pursuits. Joanna has found her own unique way to cope with her symptoms by reaching out to others.

It is worth noting that all of the individuals discussed above recognize that not everyone in their social environment can understand their needs or respond appropriately to them. In fact, they have come to learn that it is not a given that family members are their best supports. They have periodically sought out mental health professionals who can provide more objective feedback, insights, and coping strategies. They have also learned that sometimes limited "doses of exposure" to unsupportive others keep their stress levels manageable and their cognitive skills better protected. They understand that when their physical, cognitive, and emotional resources are already limited, they simply cannot afford to invest in relationships that deplete those resources.

The Role of Others for You

1. Recognize the stress-buffering and energy-conserving value of social support.
2. Talk candidly with others about your cognitive symptoms, and strategize about how others can assist you in minimizing the negative impact of those symptoms.
3. Be interpersonally selective. Avoid those who are unable to be supportive or who increase your stress and challenge your cognitive skills and endurance.
4. Consider consulting with a mental health professional as needed.

Strategy #7 Being Flexible, Open, and Able to Laugh

For individuals with chronic and/or progressive conditions, the goal of having a sense of predictability and control in one's life can be quite elusive. This is especially true in a condition like MS, but it may be particularly challenging to those individuals with MS who have a more controlling or rigid personality style. One person with MS described his condition as "God's way of teaching people with control issues that they cannot control everything." Therefore, the goal of predictability and control becomes supplanted by flexibility and openness in the face of the unknown.

Inherent in the MS experience is the idea that *who I am* and *what I do today* may not be *who I am* and *what I do tomorrow*. To navigate this slippery slope successfully, one has to be willing to modify one's approach in response to health changes. I am reminded of an analogous experience during my graduate school training in which I applied one statistical formula to all the problems on my statistics exam, when, in fact, this formula was the appropriate choice for only a few of the problems. I did poorly on the exam because I responded in one particular way to a situation calling for a variety of responses.

For the individual with MS, the openness to new strategies and accommodations, as well as increases in social supports, is essential. One needs a full array of cognitive, emotional, and physical tools, recognizing that some may do the trick some of the time and be ineffective at other times. Moreover, it means being proactive about this without painting a catastrophic picture of the future for oneself. For example, a couple may discuss how they plan to handle a future exacerbation, or may entertain possible, longer-term options for the future, should cognitive symptoms increase in their number or severity. This planning during a moment of calm is likely to be more effective and less stressful than having to make quick decisions in the midst of a crisis. Unanticipated changes will occur. Acknowledging and accepting their potential emergence allows a person to make necessary adjustments and succeed.

Marie has learned that she never knows what she is going to wake up to (with regard to her symptoms) on any given day.

She accepts that some days are going to be better than others and reminds herself regularly that life could be worse. Sarah, whenever possible, tries not to leave anything she has to do for the last minute because she cannot predict whether she will have a good or a bad day by the time her deadline approaches. Joanna describes her own letting go of the "external markers of success." The shifts she has made in her professional life have meant foregoing a promotion to full professor, yet doing it her way provided her with a rich, new source of self-esteem. Steve has moved from the technical aspects of his profession to the human side. He may no longer design medical equipment, but he is ensuring that consumers of this equipment—himself included—are getting the quality products they need. Being open to modifying their goals enabled their success in a new direction.

Humor can be a wonderful stress release after keys have been misplaced for the umpteenth time or you wonder repeatedly why you went into a particular room. The healing power of humor and laughter are documented in a number of studies.[13] For example, after exposing a group of people to a humorous situation, a pair of researchers found an increase in the number and activity level in "natural killer cells" within these people. Natural killer cells are cells that attack viral-infected cells and some kinds of cancer cells.[14] Other studies have suggested that humor has a strengthening effect on the immune system in a number of different ways.[15]

How does a person apply humor to cognitive challenges? One woman with MS talks about how her family playfully teases her about her use of primitive sign language when she experiences word-finding difficulties. They laugh together, temporarily defusing the familiar, frustrating moment. Another person with MS describes how laughing at his momentary inability to remember a name is the way he "eases up" on himself. A young teen with obsessive-compulsive disorder turns his next challenge in overcoming his excessive cleaning rituals into a fun game. He invites his family to "descend" on his room and disrupt some of its order and then allows them to playfully distract him from rushing to clean it. Finally, a girl with attention-deficit/hyperactivity disorder has a laugh with her parents as she suddenly interrupts an important conversation to comment on something interesting, but irrelevant—and then never returns to her original conversation.

Although there is no question that MS is a serious disease with significant implications for one's day-to-day and future functioning, infusing lightness through humor can make the "heaviness" of the condition more manageable and one's perspective more hopeful. And given the promising evidence on humor's impact on the immune system, laughter may prove to be good medicine in the fight against the cognitive, physical, and emotional challenges of MS.

Allowing Yourself to Be Open and Flexible

1. Educate yourself about the variety of strategies that can be used to offset cognitive symptoms such as memory deficits, distractibility, organizational difficulties, or word-finding problems.
2. Recognize that different days may call for different approaches.
3. Trade in rigid views of who you are, how you are supposed to be, and what you should be doing for more flexible, novel, even creative ways of feeling good about yourself.
4. Take time to laugh at yourself and at life, and share the humor with others.

The Role of a Careful Assessment

There are many facets to cognitive functioning. Some skills are obvious, such that we know when we possess the skills and when we don't. For example, we tend to know whether we are good organizers, spellers, or problem-solvers. Others are much more subtle, like attention to visual detail, eye-hand coordination, and cognitive flexibility (that is, how easily we can shift from one cognitive task to another).

I cannot emphasize enough the importance of evaluating cognitive strengths and limitations with a neuropsychological evaluation. This evaluation is the most comprehensive assessment of cognitive functioning and provides invaluable baseline and follow-up data about the "state of the brain" and how that state translates into functional behavior. A good neuropsychological evaluation will also include detailed recommendations for how to combat or manage cognitive deficits so that one's functioning is optimized.

As a clinical psychologist, I also cannot overlook the importance of viewing mental health as a vital ingredient in keeping cognitive skills sharp in individuals with MS or other chronic conditions. Nothing can dull the mind, spirit, and body like a depression. High levels of anxiety can immobilize and can significantly undermine skills such as attention, perception, and problem-solving.

There is some MS research to suggest that symptoms of depression or irritability seen in some people with MS may be part of an exacerbation of the disease, rather than the emotional consequence of it.[16,17,18] This speaks to the potential benefit of antidepressant medication as part of the MS treatment regimen. Likewise, it is important to psychotherapeutically treat those adjustment issues and emotional symptoms that result from having the disease, inasmuch as these issues and symptoms can overload the brain and undermine cognitive skills. When a person is immersed in sadness, helplessness, hopelessness, or the fear that a health crisis may strike at any moment, there is less room for focused or productive thinking, accurate recall of information and experiences, or overall mental clarity. Family members may also desire or need to be involved in psychotherapy to address their own adjustment difficulties or to learn how to provide the most appropriate support.

“Bit by Bit, Putting it Together”[19]

One goal of this chapter is to encourage readers to examine what personal puzzle pieces are in place as they face cognitive challenges of MS in themselves or others. Recall my discovery that I could take a piece from one puzzle and put it in the same location in another. Consider the implications of this discovery. Once I exchanged a piece, I essentially created a new puzzle.

Once you take the “pieces” described in this chapter, whether it is, for example, learning to pace oneself, playing to one’s strengths, or finding meaning in a changed life, the overall picture begins to look different. A person becomes a newly integrated entity. And while that new entity may feel less familiar to ourselves and those around us, it can work.

Joanna, the woman with posttraumatic stress disorder, talks about her journey as “a struggle to look at all the pieces on the floor and try to put them back together in some way. This is a different me, some parts recognizable, others are new. You may not recognize the whole picture any longer….Some pieces were missing and may still be missing.” The individuals in the case vignettes have made a positive transformation, and they are open to and ready for the new pieces in their lives, whether they are coping pieces or challenge pieces.

We can also use the puzzle analogy to emphasize the idea that one’s puzzle does not have to stand alone. The borrowed pieces can represent the others in our lives who fill in the missing parts. Thus, the building of the new puzzle can be an effort that is shared with your support team, and the end result can be one that is stronger and more resilient. Even when a cognitive MS exacerbation occurs and essentially “tips over the puzzle table,” having strategies at the ready makes reassembly or the building of new puzzles more possible.

In conclusion, in order to be prepared to meet the changes and challenges that go hand in hand with MS, and to preserve mental sharpness, one needs to draw on a number of important resources. One needs to view cognitive or physical changes associated with MS as only a part of one's overall identity and to shift one's focus onto the strengths that also define a person. One also needs to set reasonable goals and pursue them at a reasonable pace. This may require an individual to say "no" and set limits with family, friends, coworkers, and strangers. A person must strive to find meaning in his life even while mourning losses, protect his mental health, and recognize that the process of coping with the unpredictability of MS should not occur in a social vacuum.

Lastly, one must approach this MS journey with openness, flexibility, and humor, as the journey has its obstacles and detours. A person need not accept the picture on the MS puzzle box cover as the one that limits her life. Finding richness and beauty within the experience of any chronic disease like MS depends on one's willingness to examine one's own puzzle picture and rearrange its pieces until a more adaptive, fulfilling solution is achieved.

Mental Sharpening Stones and Perspectives

The adjustment to the diagnosis of MS and its physical and cognitive symptoms requires a shift in how a person defines herself. There is a process that moves from grieving and victimization to acceptance, integration of the new view of self, and empowerment. In order to successfully make the above transition, the following strategies are necessary.

1. Playing to One's Strengths
    - Focusing on activities that involve cognitive skills unaffected by MS
    - Avoiding excessive physical or intellectual activity to prevent fatigue and the potential for an exacerbation
    - Engaging in regular mental and physical exercise

2. Removing the Obstacles
    - Consulting with an occupational therapist regarding optimal ways of structuring home and work environments
    - Making use of organizational strategies, memory aids, and technologic advances
3. Setting Limits
    - Being selective in committing to responsibilities
    - Learning to say “no” without guilt
    - Avoiding unnecessary stress
4. Pacing
    - Programming in “guilt-free” breaks
    - Resisting the temptation to overdo or set unrealistic deadlines
    - Avoiding “multitasking”
5. Searching for Meaning
    - Seeking out experiences that are future-oriented and enhance self-esteem
    - Considering the pursuit of goals and activities long abandoned or shelved
    - Engaging in activities that transform limitations and challenges into something positive
6. Recognizing the Importance of Others
    - Recognizing the stress-buffering and energy-conserving value of social support
    - Talking candidly and strategizing with others
    - Being interpersonally selective
    - Considering consultation with a mental health professional as needed
7. Being Flexible, Open and Able to Laugh
    - Educating oneself about the variety of strategies available to minimize the impact of cognitive symptoms
    - Recognizing that different days may call for different approaches

- Trading in rigid views for more flexible, novel, even creative ways of feeling good
- Taking time to laugh and sharing the humor with others

References

1. Kübler-Ross E. *On Death and Dying*. New York: Macmillan; 1969.
2. Reitberg MB, Brooks D, Uitdehaag BMJ, Kwakkel G. Exercise therapy for multiple sclerosis. Cochrane Database Syst Rev 2005;1:CD003980; DOI:10.1002/14651858:CD003980.
3. Fensterheim H, Baer J. *Don't Say Yes When You Want to Say No*. New York: Random House; 1975.
4. Smith MJ. *When I Say No I Feel Guilty*. New York: Bantam; 1985.
5. Birnbaum P, translator. *Ethics of the Fathers: Pirke Avot*. Whitefish, MT: Kessinger Publishing; 2007.
6. Catanzaro M, Kraft GH. *Living with Multiple Sclerosis: a Wellness Approach*, 2nd ed. New York: Demos Medical Publishing; 2000.
7. Frankl VE. *Man's Search for Meaning*. New York: Washington Square Press; 1959.
8. See for example: Shapiro F, Forrest MS. *EMDR: The Breakthrough Therapy for Overcoming Anxiety, Stress and Trauma*. New York: Basic Books, 1997.
9. *Diagnostic and Statistical Manual of Mental Disorders*, 4th ed. Washington: American Psychiatric Association; 1994.
10. Cobb S. Social support as a moderator of life stress. *Psychosom Med* 1976;38(5):300-314.
11. Thoits PA. Stress, coping and social support processes: Where are we? What next? *J Health Soc Behavior* 1995;35:53-79.
12. Clinton HR. *It Takes a Village*. New York: Simon & Schuster; 1996.
13. Fry WF. The physiologic effects of humor, mirth and laughter. *JAMA* 1992;267(13):1857-1858.
14. Berk L, Tan S. Eustress of mirthful laughter modifies natural killer cell activity. *Clin Res* 1989;37:115.

15. Dillon KM, Minchoff B, Baker KH. Positive emotional states and enhancement of the immune system. *Int J Psychiatry* 1985-1986;15(1):13-18.

16. *Depression and Multiple Sclerosis*, a brochure. New York: National Multiple Sclerosis Society; 2007.

17. Pujol J, Bello J, Deus J, Marti-Vilalta JL, Capdevila A. Lesions in the left arcuate fasciculus region and depressive symptoms in multiple sclerosis. *Neurology* 1997;49(4):1105-1110.

18. Schubert DS, Foliart RH. Increased depression in multiple sclerosis patients: a meta-analysis. *Psychosomatics* 1993;34(2):124-130.

19. Sondheim S. *Putting It Together*. From “Sunday in the Park with George.” New York: RCA Records; 1984.

CHAPTER 6

The Dance of Life: Transformation to Maintaining Strength, Balance, and Focus

Carol Crawford Smith

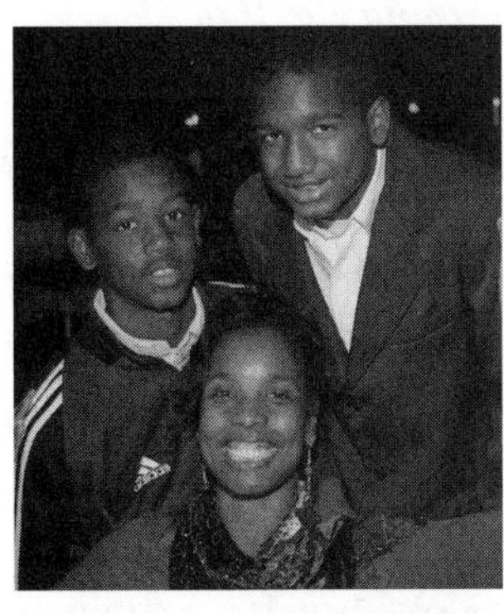

Carol Crawford Smith is a former ballerina of the Dance Theatre of Harlem. She has a Master of Science degree in Human Development from Virginia Tech and is Founder and Artistic Director of The Center of Dance in Blacksburg, Virginia. In 2006, she and her children were featured recipients on the ABC television show "Extreme Makeover: Home Edition."

For an artist of any form, it is instinctual to bring a creative element into every engagement or ordinary activity. This may include cooking and eating a flavorful and colorful meal to stacking groceries in a cart in a balanced and aesthetically pleasing formation. It is instinctual for the artist to formulate things, situations, and circumstances so that they are meaningful and attractive, leaving the observer, recipient, or oneself feeling enlightened and empowered from the experience. In that light, it is the intention of this writing to invite the reader to learn how it is possible, through exploring cognitive creation, to continue to produce excellence in a profession and passion when physical limitations could dictate the contrary.

This is also a conversation about dis-ease that has manifested in my life and body. It's a conversation that I have been avoiding, not wanting to deal with the pain involved in coming to terms with truth. Now, I do so willingly and openly. One truth is that I no longer dance because of increasing and seemingly irreversible physical disability from multiple sclerosis (MS). However, because I do not dance with my body anymore, and I am a dance teacher now, I have embraced the importance of developing and maintaining movement through thought. Maintaining mental strength has enabled me to remain a dancer and continue in the profession, as long as I keep my mind active and sharp. It is like every day taking a cognitive dance class with the realization of how vital maintaining the thought component is to my profession and everything else I do.

Each New Day

Like most others, the morning is greeted with words of thanks for being alive another day and for the new breaths taken. "Thank you for this day and for the breath of life," I say quietly. Upon awakening, I remain still in bed to analyze my physical ability for the moment. "Is using a walker or a wheelchair best?" I question. But before doing anything, I must figure out how to maneuver my spastic and stiff body up to a sitting position from having lain flat and sedate the entire night.

Not many go through such complex thought processes and actions upon awakening. Most people simply roll over, stand to their feet, and shuffle to the bathroom with eyes barely open. Not me. I am wide awake upon reaching a sitting position on the edge of the mattress. Once I have decided whether to travel via foot or wheels, other activities for the morning are already planned. "Okay, go to the bathroom and then go get some water," I say to myself. "And before getting a drink, see if there is a load of washing or drying that can be started."

My laundry facilities are located between the master bedroom and bathroom. It makes sense to do a chore while passing through to efficiently use morning time and energy. Both resources are precious and few these days. Time is valued because it is a momentary gift in which actions take place. Energy is vital because it is essential for producing the actions. Both are now compromised and encumbered because of a condition I endure.

The condition used to be labeled "a challenge," more specifically as "a health challenge." How is it described now? Frankly, there are no good labels or descriptive adjectives. If anyone questions my use of a wheelchair, my response is, "I was diagnosed with MS." The reaction is sometimes doom and gloom followed with, "But you are so young and so beautiful," or "It is great that you keep going." Well daahh, somehow I missed the memo that reported MS meant an ugly inactive life. Anyone who expects me to be a feeble and incognizant MS patient ultimately sees a young woman diagnosed with the disease who is raising two sons, runs her own business, and remains quite active in society and life. This is the outward appearance. Seen from within is the woman who has come to say, "Thank you for this 'gift' and its humbling effect that causes me to develop into a more powerful and generous human being." Now don't get me wrong. I would summon the gratitude, and return the "gift" in a heartbeat, then keep the power and generous spirit for a lifetime!

✻ The "Gift" Arrives

I am the Founder and Artistic Director of a dance school, The Center of Dance. In the fall of 1999, after producing, directing, choreographing, and performing in two major stage events, I was simply worn out. The fatigue kept increasing, and my body and energy would not recover even after taking the usual measures to rest and recuperate. By December 31st, I had a routine medical check-up. Blood tests were ordered to see if something "funky" was going on inside. The night after the appointment, there was a distinct discomfort in my left side. It was prominent in the neck and progressed through the shoulder and arm and down through my hand. My fingers were quite numb and weak as well. The intensity subsided but never fully dissipated. To this day, I still have numbness and stiffness in my left hand that has leapt over to the right, and my left shoulder stiffens severely on a cold day.

Y2K hit. In mid-January, after a winter break, it was time to return to the studio and begin teaching for the new season. As a dancer who owns and operates a dance business, ballet is my forte and my first dance love. It is not uncommon for a dancer to be exceptionally good at ballet but hate it with no reservations because it is a technique that requires perfection and exactness, yet can never be perfected. Doing it can lead to constant dissatisfaction if the expectation to be perfect exists. From the "doer" to the viewer, there is always going to be criticism that can cause frustration. In spite of this truth, I simply love ballet. I love the way it feels to do it, and I do not care what anyone thinks or says about it! That was until I could not physically dance anymore.

The euphoric feeling of dancing comes especially when taking ballet class or performing. This is probably why the love is so strong because 99% of being a dancer is about studying and physically honing, perfecting, and displaying the technique. The remaining 1% is a private "aha moment" that only the dancer knows.

"Okay, let's begin!" I enthusiastically call all dancers to collect for the beginning of class. Everyone had a place at the barre, including me at the helm to demonstrate the first combination. "First position. Port de bras, one and two," I simultaneously call out the combination and do it. By now, everyone was familiar with the standard warm up. When I demonstrate the combination with the students, it reinforces what they already know, while giving me a chance to work out. If anyone were new to a class on any given day, the person would simply follow along as I proceeded to do combinations on the right and then on the left side at the barre.

My reason and objective for opening the studio is met with every class taught. It is the insatiable desire to dance forever. With each class taught, the dream is compounded and the objective met through relaying the steps verbally, physically, and spiritually. All I have to do is hear the music. Sometimes just hearing one or two bars is sufficient to formulate a combination. The vision of the movement is internally seen and felt when the beat and rhythm are heard. My mind knows what to do with the music and instantly tells my body how it should move.

At the peak of my physical capabilities, the body would become the music. It would instinctively flow and move with and in the rhythm. On top of the instinct was the applied knowledge of the correct progressive format for a dance class. A ballet class, for example, would begin with the plié or the bending of the knees to warm up the legs, stretch the Achilles, and control turnout from the hips. Accompanying the legwork is a coordinated or held arm movement called the port de bras. Together, the upper and lower body render a pose or a moving picture of beauty and grace that can excite the viewer and the doer to a point of physical prowess or ecstasy.

Ballet is the foundation of my professional dance career, but I absolutely enjoy and relate to just about all forms of dance. At that first week of returning to teaching, I demonstrated a combination in a jazz class and landed a jeté leap on a collapsed right leg. "Tombé pas de bourre, glissade jeté, jeté, jeté…," I called out the combination while demonstrating. The leap was executed with typical height, flexibility, and strength. The landing was met with weakness and lack of control. There was no way of pretending that what just happened was a simple mishap that could be played off and worked through. Something was undeniably wrong.

Upon the next day's return to the studio to teach morning ballet, my body still felt weak and uncomfortable. Leg strength and movement control were diminished and compromised. The feeling was incomprehensible and my confidence was rattled. I was baffled by the feelings of numbness and weakness and began to tear up in front of the class of adult women. What in the world was going on? My body was simply not acting right! My memory knew exactly every component of the technique, but the muscles were clearly not following instructions that seem to be left in my mind. No matter how much I internally questioned, got frustrated, or reasoned that the situation should be to the contrary, the condition was not budging.

It is still difficult to describe or imagine. It was as if some foreign entity had taken over me physically, and it was in control of my body. As a dancer, my body was my instrument. Daily tuning and conditioning through exercise and dance technique class was what I depended on to maintain my gorgeous, contoured, strong, and graceful physique. But things were all out of whack. At that very moment, I felt like I was in a struggle for survival of the only life known. "Stop it!" An internal order sounded. Not wanting to suffer in silence, I stopped the class to rehash and talk through what I was feeling and the order of events that transpired. At the close of explaining, I downplayed and simplified the present feeling as a "pinched" nerve.

"If it's a 'pinched' nerve, all you have to do is un-pinch it," one student remarked.

"Yeah," I reasoned and wanted to believe the solution was that simple. She went on to say it sounded like more than a pinched nerve and suggested a visit to a neurologist. Since the woman was the wife of a doctor, her recommendation was respected and an appointment was scheduled.

On February 2, 2000, I was sitting in a consultation room with the attending neurologist. He proceeded to explain the magnetic resonance images taken of my brain and spine as if reciting from a textbook. I understood the dialogue and made the correlation between the white masses seen in the image to the word "plaques" used to describe them. He proceeded to say terms needing more explanation such as "myelin sheaths," and eventually stated a very foreign term.

"It looks like multiple sclerosis," were his exact words. He labeled it the probable diagnosis.

"What in the world is multiple sclerosis?" was my immediate reaction. "Am I going to die?" was my second question.

"No," he snickered. Thoughts of my children began racing in my head. My youngest son had just turned four and my oldest son was six. I would not tell them what had transpired at the doctor's office, since the boys were too young to understand. Heck, I did not even fully understand.

The way to deal with it was to not show that anything was different. There would be no emotional outbursts and no disruptions in activities of daily living. All would be normal and business as usual. Mommy would take them to the park to kick balls, climb on jungle gyms, and swing on swings. Teaching dance would continue without question. It was necessary. The income from the dance school paid for studio operations, family health insurance, groceries, gas for the car, and clothes and shoes for growing boys. Teaching could not be forfeited. Besides, I needed to teach to dance forever!

The Journey to Eternal Dancing

In October 1978, I began my professional dance career with the Dance Theatre of Harlem (DTH). Although I was still in high school, the company directors invited me to live in New York City and work with the company. Little did I know that I had committed to a chance of a lifetime with an internationally renowned performing arts ensemble. In the beginning of that period, I completed preparatory education and graduated from Professional

Children's School with honors, while living in an apartment on my own. I traveled via subway or bus to and from school, the company headquarters, and home on a daily basis. Weekends were spent riding Metro North up the Hudson to my hometown of Poughkeepsie. The rest of my time was spent touring the world to places I had only once imagined.

What began as eight daily hours for six days a week of ballet classes and rehearsals in a studio on the second floor of a renovated fire station turned into a decade-long career of performances in world-famous opera houses such as Covent Garden in London; the Mariyinski Theatre in Saint Petersburg (then Leningrad), Russia; the Metropolitan Opera House in NYC; and the Kennedy Center in Washington, DC.

My career with DTH was phenomenal. It was an unparalleled experience that afforded me the opportunity to be in performances enjoyed by global luminaries such as Her Royal Highness Princess Diana, President and Mrs. Ronald Reagan, prima ballerinas Margot Fontayne and Lynn Seymour, and danseurs étoile Rudolph Nureyev and Mihail Baryshnikov. I spoke intimately with them about dancing and learned of the delight they received seeing the performance.

Even with all of the exterior wonder, the real joy and satisfaction came from the work and commitment to create a body that was pure pleasure and magical to live in. On a sweltering hot summer day we, the DTH company would open the fire-escape door of the studio to welcome a breeze of warm air. Dancers were seen pirouetting in puddles of perspiration without slipping. To successfully do this meant the reward of fine-tuning balance, strengthening muscles for suspension, and developing the greatest body control. All of this proficiency was especially useful when accomplishing an exceptional performance, which occurred in the south of France during a summer arts festival.

The arena was an outdoor amphitheater in Arles. It began to rain one evening while we were performing, and a cool chill in the air caused the wet stage floor to freeze a bit, presenting a challenge to dance on. The show went on. At the height of the cold, wet, and frozen conditions, I had to execute a series of quick and precise pirouettes on pointe, as if turning on a dime. Calling heavily on the control and ability to suspend through the torso and lengthen out of the standing leg, I successfully completed the series with no break or fall.

This same control developed from years of dance training was relied on heavily when the MS diagnosis came and muscle weakness began. I instinctively walk in a rhythm and move to music like nobody's business. Now movement is cumbersome. It is stiff and laborious. Where I once flowed like a willow in the wind and maintained balance for many counts, I now remain as stagnant as a piece of petrified redwood and cannot stand on my own, let alone upright for more than a split second. All of my dance technique still thrives in my thoughts but remains disconnected from the fine use of my body with no clear direction or end. So now, after 13 years of dancing in New York and 13 more years of enjoying the art through my business, I find myself with the diagnosis of an unwanted debilitating disease.

A Lonely Road

What's in a name? This is a question frequently asked when reasoning the "where, when, why, and what" of the diagnosis of MS. My ex-husband was with me when the disease was diagnosed (interestingly, his initials are M.S.), and, after learning the diagnosis, we left the doctor's office together.

"Now it's my turn to get my career in order!" he angrily ranted on the way to the parking lot. Scared and confused, I wondered why he was so mad at me. Feeling guilty, responsible, and incompetent all at once, I felt I had let him down by getting sick. His response and reaction were dumbfounding. There was absolutely no comfort or consoling from him. He got in his car and drove off in a hurried huff, leaving me devastated, feeling alone, and not knowing what to do or say.

In a case such as this, one turns to God like never before. I prayed during the entire lone drive home and asked, then begged, and ultimately pleaded with God to take the symptoms away and make me normal. I began to read the Bible and spiritual journals and publications regularly in search of answers and understanding. God was the One to turn to for comfort, as my mate demonstrated he neither could nor would be there for me emotionally or physically. From then on, I consciously did not complain or fret about the numbness or nagging discomfort that persisted, nor did I openly discuss the diagnosis or my understanding of it. Discussing the situation meant paying it attention and giving it power to exist. My belief was that if the words multiple sclerosis were not articulated and the concept ignored, it would all simply release and vanish.

This mindset developed from years of conditioning as a ballerina to envision only what you wish to achieve as well as to never complain, show weakness, or admit anything is ever wrong. Even if performing a ballet on pointe with raw and blistered feet, wrenched knees, and Achilles riddled with tendonitis, a ballerina must remain poised at all times and not allow the audience to see the person behind the character or pain. The illusionary life of the ballerina was ingrained. Not once did the characterization of an autoimmune disease infiltrate into my world, and I was stubbornly determined not to perform the role now. It was time to be a diva, cut those rehearsals, and forfeit being cast in the starring role of the "disease production" of MS.

More importantly, it was time to stop living the illusionary life of being happily married and in a stable and nurturing relationship. Not owning up to this reality for nearly a decade was emotionally, physically, and spiritually draining. From here came my first lesson and steps on how to cognitively recreate my life and deal with my health. I had to be honest about my marital situation and the psychological and emotional abuse that I had suffered. I had to think through, recap, and own up to the order of events that led to the diagnosis. Once identified and acknowledged, the culprits had to be eliminated from my life.

Establishing and Maintaining Normalcy within the Admission of Truth

I admitted that my husband could not be depended upon to support my children and me. I had to determine how to take care of us without him. My patience was spent, and there was no time to enable his incompetence any longer. Once squashed in an abusive domestic relationship, I was breaking through full force with no hesitation or apprehension. It was necessary to reinvent myself and be the phenomenally independent and able woman that I truly am.

My immediate truth and dream was to be a homeowner. I began looking for a house for my sons and me to live in. In the process, thoughts of having an unfamiliar disease regularly crept into my conscious. The concerns were ignored and I carried on. The one constant thought, concern, or dis-ease, if you will, that persisted was the ugly communications and circumstances of the MS that I had lived with for the previous 10 years. That part of those years was filled with stress, unhappiness, and uncertainty, not knowing whether there would be a stable income to live on or a roof over my head to call my own. I ignored that reality for so long and just would not admit it to be true. In writing, I see the parallel of the dis-ease of my marriage and the disease of my body. It is painful to see but so freeing to admit. The refusal to say the words multiple sclerosis or read or listen to anything about the disease continued to be my resolve and my way to deal with things. I chose to not focus on MS and began releasing MS.

In my not focusing on MS, anger and resentment showed their face anytime someone mentioned the diagnosis. It seemed like everybody and their mother came to me with stories of someone they knew affected, if they did not have it themselves. When this happened, I quickly diverted the focus of the conversation. The last thing I wanted to talk about was how I was feeling and start a pity party. Listening to or telling "woe is me" stories was most definitely out of the question.

I once let my guard down and confidentially mentioned the diagnosis to the mother of a student. Upon being told, she hissed and pulled back as if I had the plague. Her actions read like "Don't touch me! I don't want to catch it!" The reaction was heart wrenching. People always wanted to get close to me and be in my presence. At that moment, I felt like an outcast. From then on, a sturdier shield of silence and denial was lifted as protection against who was told.

As news of the diagnosis spread to my dancers and into the community at large, I carried on as if it could be worked through and would soon pass. Classes and rehearsals continued. There were performances to produce and commitments to fulfill. I continued to work long and hard hours teaching, maintaining records, and doing public relations and all other entrepreneurial duties, believing it necessary to maintain independence and to live.

Dance to Live

Dance is my life and performing was essential to living. The last time I performed on stage was February 12, 2000, in a work I choreographed entitled *UJIMA Heat*. One section of the dance requires balancing on the right leg for five steady measures of six. My right leg was stronger, but the left had to remain involved. I made it through the sequence with concern and doubt while doing, then continued on through the fast section of the dance. Onto the end, the cast of five worked toward center stage and ended in a dramatic finale pose. STAGE BLACK. An ironic lighting cue to end the piece, as I have not danced in a performance since then.

This was the first and last time I relied predominantly on cognitive recollection and direction to physically get through a dance, since I was not completely feeling what I was doing. There was no sure way to know if the movements were happening correctly. My body did not function automatically or reflexively as usual, so my mind had to kick into full-control mode to make things happen and be totally focused on the physical detail.

Before the MS diagnosis and symptoms set in, the use of thought to make the body function was taken for granted. Use of thought just happened when dancing and I simply didn't realize it. Movement was natural and reflexive. Doesn't thinking make this so? I'd hear the music and would feel the rhythm, and my body would respond as instinctively as a heartbeat. Since my body is slowed now, the same music and beats are felt mentally. I literally close my eyes or allow them to remain open to "see—but don't see" and move my brain to the beats, then formulate the words and actions for the steps.

Once the terms are identified, the directive of what to dance was given to my body. And now the same approach is used to teach steps to my students. I engage the precise memories of skill, dance in the mind, and explain the movements. Words are formulated from the thought-generated feelings to articulate the spirit and mechanics of dancing. Maintaining my physical strength and ability, as well as verbally relaying body applications to other people, established for me a direct cognitive connection to the physical part. Each depends on the other.

I do not take a step now when even walking without thinking about how my feet are placed, where my knees are pointed, or if my shoulders are hunched and compromised for balance. And I do not give a combination or move to my students without crafting the most appropriate collection of words to relay so they know exactly what steps to do. Even with learning simple motion, conveying accurate detail in the instruction is key to instilling the correct movement.

Walking is my gift to me, and it is highly valued. Like dancing, walking is instinctual and second nature. "Walking is dancing," I tell students. "When you walk down the street, you do not bring the same arm forward as leg. No, you walk in opposition. The right arm goes forward with the left leg and vice versa with each step taken." I always tell this to my students, especially when teaching them to coordinate their steps and positions.

Dance is about coordination and opposition. For example, a basic position such as tendu croisé (ton-DEW krwah-ZAY) is executed on an X-axis. The leg is crossed front or back of the body center with the arms extended above or beyond the shoulders to expand or accentuate the chest and torso. The head and shoulders then take the lead of the body to create complimentary épaulmente. Croisé is very open in the upper body but private in the lower half. Again, the concept of opposition is expressed to produce proper ballet technique. As I verbally explain what I can no longer demonstrate with my body, students understand. My approach has been successful, and I've learn to appreciate the vital cognitive aspect of dance, as I experienced with one student named Lucy.

Mental Dance with Lucy

Lucy has been studying with me since she was five years old. She began in the Fundamentals of Dance class, where children are encouraged to move freely at one point and then in an organized fashion to properly execute the steps and movements. Lucy knows me as a dancer, as well as her teacher. She has seen me perform both in class and on stage. Her demeanor was often coy as a small child, acting shy and frightened, sometimes hiding behind a classmate when the class was called to the center of the studio to perform combinations.

As years progressed, Lucy's confidence developed and I frequently called her forward to demonstrate. In those years, her teacher changed. Lucy was about 12 when my physical debilitation became obvious. It was difficult for me physically and emotionally to go to the studio and teach. So, for a good dance year, I barely taught at all but ran the business from my home. Classes kept going with the assistance of dancers and instructors in the community who came forward to help. They heard my health was not good and that I was considering closing the school. The community was concerned, and talented instructors offered to teach classes in my absence to give me a chance to rest and think about what I would do.

Through this time, Lucy stayed. I was no longer her regular teacher, her pillar of dance strength, but my spirit was vibrant within the studio walls, and she remained faithful. Now in high school, Lucy is a beautiful, self-assured sophomore who has progressed on to the study of pointe. Pointe work is demanding and difficult and requires great strength and control. Lucy successfully carried on the teaching learned in her early years of study and is now a strong ballet dancer performing solo pointe variations.

Recently, when teaching a ballet class, I gave Lucy corrections and pointers to improve her technique. She did not hesitate to respectfully tell me that her now-regular instructor requests something a little different. Oh, the ego flags went flying high inside my head. How dare she stand up there and tell me she is taught to do something different now?! I admired her though for speaking up and was reminded of my own encouragement for dancers to seek instruction from other teachers and take the best of the lesson that works for them without negating the fundamentals. She had learned well outside of my guidance, and I had to accept letting my dance baby go to fly on her own.

The very next day, I observed Lucy in class doing a similar position as the one corrected the day before. Guess what? It was perfected using the influence of both the current teacher and me. How proud I was to see that she took what was given and made it work within the parameters of correct technique. Just as dance is my life, I also learned to let others find their existence in dance.

I no longer jump up and show people what a position or movement looks like and insist that they do it my way. Instead, I describe the attitude associated with the technique and hope it will register.

When Lucy was in my class, she was exaggerating the épaulmante (ay-pohl-MAHN) to the point of having too much arch in her back. "Lucy," I said, "lift your chest and back to have the correct incline and tilt of the upper body and head. Do not stick out your ribs and butt to form a collapsed duck-like position." The other instructor was teaching the dancers more advanced épaulmente or proper use of head and shoulders when in ballet positions. This instruction is quite appropriate for Lucy's current level of learning, but, what I was seeing on Lucy, was an affectation or stylized idea of what the teacher was saying to do. The concept was there, but it was unsuccessfully accomplished to the point where it could be harmful to her body if continued. I calmly described the proper positioning for the technique, and Lucy successfully adapted. The outcome was a win-win situation for all involved.

From the case of mentally guiding Lucy to apply correct technique, there is assurance that my ability to verbally articulate dance positions is effective for getting students to understand and apply correct technique without me personally providing a physical example to model. In some ways, my not providing the physical example is even more effective. The dancers are not focused on the visual example and pigeonholed into doing exactly as I do but can hear my expert advice and take from it what works best for their personal achievement and accomplishment. By keeping my mind focused on the particulars of movement to share with others, I felt my spirit performing with her.

I am grateful to the individuals who took over teaching in my absence eight years ago. Their assistance enabled the doors to remain open while I refocused and recommitted and was of a better mindset and position to return to teaching using a honed gift of verbal articulation and detailed mental guidance. MS has not erased my ability to know proper dance technique. To the contrary, my understanding has been perfected. By expressing and exercising movements mentally, the delivery is formulated and a connection is made to others through verbal instruction. As a ballet instructor who shares dance through detailed mental guidance, my skill, balance, and focus in the art form remain strong—I still dance.

New Performance Mediums

It's been eight years since I last danced on stage or showed a movement in class. I initially missed the ability to physically perform for an audience and demonstrate steps to my students. Eventually, I saw the blessing in it because I truly needed a break. Through the years, hope remains that the symptoms are temporary and will one day pass with the awakening of a completely disease-free body. Such thoughts help maintain focus on the things I can control and ward off depression and anxiety. Life is different now and, in some ways, quite the same.

Today, eight years since the diagnosis, my association with MS is exposed publicly through writings, social forums, and television broadcasts. Such extensive exposure was vehemently rejected in the past, mainly due to me wanting to preserve the crafted image of a poised, graceful, and in-control individual with no apparent weakness or incompetence. As I become more comfortable with my disposition, I seize beneficial opportunities to perform in a new voice, which includes sharing my dance expertise and remaining mentally connected to dance technique by examining the detail of what my body knows instinctively and relating it verbally. It's as if I have done a grande jeté (big throw leap) over MS, turned around, and gave it a grande battement (big kick) in the seat of its pants. In others words, MS has not got the best of me.

Whether writing, speaking publicly, or simply going about daily living, I no longer harbor fear of what others will think when seeing me. The vision of graceful beauty perseveres and persists through a glorious life of dance, via instruction. Now when I openly talk about MS, it is like having auditioned and being cast in the role of one who realizes that others can learn from her shared example. And, I willingly share my story productively sans exploitation.

Throughout the process of writing this chapter, I take breaks to collect my thoughts or go off to accomplish more tasks of the day. Before one break, I thought about my situation and story and was inspired to walk. In fact, I walked publicly in front of my housekeeper. This is something I had not done before because of stubborn pride and fear of her reaction. I had conjured up her seeing me struggle to take steps and being disappointed and disgusted to see the site. But I reasoned that the poised and graceful ballerina still exists in my mind and spirit. There was no excuse for me to not summon that being and get off my fanny and walk a couple of steps no matter what it feels or looks like.

Like the croise in dance, much of my life is lived on an X-axis. I am a public personality and know most of the community through my dance business, church activities, and other social functions. I guess I was fooling myself almost a decade ago to believe that the diagnosis of MS could be kept private. When it became fruitless to hide and deny the symptoms, I agreed to tap into the strength and dignity I possess and allow something positive to come of it all. So, I walk now in front of people, learning not to be self-conscious and seeing the act as an inspirational performance that motivates observers to work through their own challenges and limitations—and to overcome them.

Extreme Transformation

Unequivocally, one of the smartest and healthiest decisions I made was to branch out on my own and buy a home for my sons and me to live in. It was more important than ever to have stability when I made the choice. The house was simple, yet affordable, and it was mine. The children had their own rooms, and I had the comfort of knowing there was a secure and permanent place to raise them. The house was in the same school district that my children had been attending. Although MS may have removed some control, I would not give it power to take attention away from my children and what I needed to do to provide a good home and life for them and me.

It was crucial for them to have normalcy in their lives and for activities to remain as uninterrupted as possible. I was physically in a bad state, and symptoms persisted ruthlessly at the time of the move. In fact, the condition and symptoms were feeling worse, and it was compounded by the stress and turmoil of divorce and child-custody proceedings. Not yet divorced, my soon to be ex-husband moved out of state. The move was a huge relief from the daily conflict and confusion but left me with the sole responsibility of raising two growing boys, which included coordinating school, sports, and social activities, along with running my home and dance school. On top of it all, I had to manage my health. My parents and plenty of caring people in the community offered to assist me with domestic needs, but I hesitated to call for help too frequently because I did not want to rely on others long-term to raise my sons and take care of me. I persevered with no complaint, and it had little to do with the ballerina conditioning to be content. The independence was welcome and I was overjoyed to be free to define the terms of my life.

Emotionally, life was in a good state, but, physically, there was increasingly great difficulty. Going anywhere became more and more uncomfortable. I began using one cane to walk, then two. Climbing stairs was especially difficult. There were stairs to negotiate in my home in any given location, from the front to the back door, to the multiple levels in the main living area, and to the basement to use the washer and dryer. It got to the point where I would coach the children in that chore. By then, they were ages 9 and 11.

Activities outside of the home included shopping for groceries, making trips to the gas station, and driving to just about anywhere I needed or wanted to go. What was frustrating was the increased time it took to do anything or go anywhere. As it became more and more necessary to use assistive devices to function in the day, I began to organize my time around coordinating access to canes, walkers, and wheelchairs, which included asking others to meet me at a destination and help with the transition.

It is important to note here that I could and can still drive without special mechanisms. It was getting from the car to the destination building or event that was always in question. *How would I feel once I arrived and parked the car? Would I be able to step out and walk to where needing to go? Would people be watching or would someone come to help?* This kind of chatter went on in my head just about each and every time I went out in public. Sometimes I would go to a grocery store at the other side of town or in a neighboring town, where there may be fewer people who knew me to see the struggle. When it was time to go to the studio though, there was no hiding. Parking was first come first serve on the street. Wherever I parked, I would have to walk to the building and then up 23 stairs to get to my studio and teach class.

One evening when going to teach, I had cut time close for arrival and felt rushed. Fortunately, the parking space I found was directly across the street from the building entrance. The arrival time was at a peak traffic hour. After getting out of the car, I leaned against the car to collect my confidence and wait until traffic was low enough to cross the street. When an opportune time came, I began the transition. With one cane in each hand, I moved and stepped in a coordinated manner consciously applying the dance rule of opposition known so well.

It was a hot day and my body began to stiffen and grow numb from the heat and anxiety produced by my actions. My mind told my body that it was okay to step, and it did, but midway in crossing the road, a step was taken and the connection of foot to the asphalt did not register. There was no feeling or sense of balance, and I fell right in the middle of the street. On the way down, I looked left and saw that traffic was at least four cars backed up. A friend came running from one of the cars and another friend appeared from somewhere else. Both of them helped me get to my feet and to the other side of the road.

I was not embarrassed by what occurred and dragged myself into the building and up the stairs. Once inside the studio, I simply wanted to make it to the registration desk and sit. How frustrated I felt and was simply tired of the disease and the unpredictable outcomes of functioning. "Why was this happening to me?" I did not ask this often but wanted to know. It just did not make sense. Without an answer, I went on to teach and to forget the traffic-stopping fall that had occurred.

More often than before, people began assisting me from my car to the studio and vice-versa. Just about every Thursday, Jane, the mother of one of my students would arrive at the same time to meet me before her daughter's class. She would help me in the building, up the stairs, and into the studio. She was very dedicated to her children and greatly involved in all aspects of their activities. On one particular day, she asked for permission to film her daughter, while taking class, to capture some childhood memories. This was fine by me, and I did not think anymore about it. About three months later, she and another friend approached me and told me why video footage was taken previously. Jane had solicited other dance parents and members of the community to write letters in support of me receiving the *Oprah's Wildest Dreams Come True* prize in some capacity. Well, word reached another friend, Robin, who went to Jane with the suggestion for me to apply for *Extreme Makeover: Home Edition*. Together they approached me with the idea. I was hesitant to apply, for not wanting my personal life to be on public display.

"I don't know about that," was my response when asked.

"Get over it!" Robin brandished. "You need help, and these people can help you." I hemmed and hawed a little bit and then agreed, figuring—what have I got to lose? From that moment forward, I had to let it all go. There was no room for the ego to control things or to be guarded. I had to disclose my entire personal adult history. They asked questions about everything from the names of past boyfriends, to the number of marriages I've had, banking and investment accounts, bankruptcies, and the names of my favorite color and flower.

The most important question they asked was *why* I felt I deserved a makeover. My answer was simple and direct—I am a dancer who teaches dance and I have become disabled. The diagnosis is MS, and the disability has made it increasingly difficult to function in my home or go to my place of business to work. My life was totally exposed and it was suddenly okay. I did not care anymore who knew intimate details about me. I willingly and freely exposed my entire life on paper applications, in video footage and legal contracts, and ultimately on world-wide television.

Miraculously, we were awarded the extreme makeover, and, in case you are wondering, it was and is phenomenally fantastic and fabulous. It truly is life transforming and far better than the unwelcomed makeover from MS. To have a brand new home and renovated dance studio, especially designed for my access, is the most amazing gift. What's more amazing is how more than 4000 people from the community and beyond galvanized to build and make the dream of a new home and improved life come true. Heartwarming stories of how people came together out of love and care for my children and me continue to come my way. People who did not know me, but had heard my story, drove from miles around the region as well as out of state to contribute. It is all truly amazing and still feels like it happened just yesterday! To think, it was the story of me being a person with MS that attracted the ABC network to "cast" me as the recipient.

The crew was absolutely wonderful and most accommodating throughout the entire extravaganza. Star designers Ty Pennington, Paige Hemmis, Paul DiMeo, and Preston Sharp were a pleasure to get to know. They made time fun when being filmed and shared in conversations of the heart when off tape. The ABC production cast and crew claimed us as family from then on. Ty added a very special touch to my studio that will always remind me of him and the life-changing adventure. His mother was a dancer and owned a dance studio when he was growing up. When he learned my family was being awarded the extreme makeover and that my studio would be his "special project," he consulted with his mother, Yvonne Pennington, who contributed a quote that is painted on the wall of my studio. It reads, "To dance is to connect to the divine in yourself and all humankind."

To me, this suggests that dance is an act that unifies all involved on a kindred spiritual level. It is true—her connection with dance is shared by me and now passes to my students. By maintaining the dance connection within me, through a cognitive exploration of my passion, I continue to be bonded with others. I have always experienced this truth in the dance world, and I now know it with my ABC family and in a greater capacity with my extended local family.

The building contractors and crew under the leadership of Bob Fetzer, President of Building Specialists, Inc., made sure I was cared for in the transition from old to new. They followed up on legal work, warranties, and punch-list items well over a year after the build, and, even with the building warranty expired, Bob Fezter remains a gracious and caring individual who checks on us from time to time to say hello and see that all is well. I am eternally grateful to each and every one who had anything to do with the extreme home and studio makeover. They have inspired and encouraged me to continue dancing.

The producers of ABC contacted Montel Williams when they were considering me for the award because of his MS diagnosis and the work he does to find a cure. To my surprise, he agreed to participate without hesitation and presented me with substantial funds to help pay some expenses of my dance studio. Montel's contribution, along with those of thousands of others, made it possible for me to stay in personal and professional operation in renovated accessible accommodations at work and home. Whether it is through dance or persevering through a chronic disease, we are all indeed divinely connected.

To continue my mental connection to instruction, I realize that maintaining my own body strength has a cognitive component. Similar to the ballet class ethic that I learned for my strength, flexibility, and grace, I will not let my mind fall out of shape or use. Happily, my mental sense of dance has not been severed by MS, and, hopefully, it will not be unless I let it occur through disuse. I am convinced this expertise will endure, as long as I use the knowledge and instruct with the fine details in my mind, connecting with verbal instruction to others.

This could not occur without the Makeover extravaganza, which created accessibility and the ability for me to continue. It is the greatest miracle to happen to me. Yet, while it was all occurring, I wished there was some magic wand that could be waved or a bag of tricks to find a miraculous cure for MS and the devastating effects of the disease. More than anything, people with MS want to be cured. Until that time is here, by easing my mind from concerns about access and injury, my thoughts are strong and free to leap with students in their performances and function more comfortably with a beating heart and a mind that moves to the dance of life.

Mental Sharpening Stones and Perspectives

1. From awakening to a new day to functioning through the symptoms and effects of MS, thought is constantly used for direction and actions to take to function through the day. Mentally think and reason through each action and give yourself directions to efficiently use time, energy, and physical resources to function effectively.
2. An action may have to be felt through rhythm or seen through internal vision or imagination in order to describe or identify the action. If conditions do not allow you to physically execute a desired action, then trust other senses to guide thought and dictate the movement, then verbally communicate what is to be achieved.
3. Trust and respond to the inner voice that says to stop and think through feelings and experiences. If a feeling is incomprehensible and you cannot figure out what to do, then ask yourself or others for suggestions or direction. Formulate your thoughts to describe the feelings or order of events, and then openly receive perspectives and answers from others.
4. We can see our bodies or actions as an object or thing. Envision metaphors to tell your body what it should feel and look like. As importantly, know the contrast, and formulate words to describe both the desire and the contrary, to paint a full picture of what is felt or seen to ultimately achieve it.
5. It can be painful to admit that things are wrong—physically and personally. Eventually, you move beyond denial. When you are ready to accept and be honest about the situation, use thought to separate illusion from actuality. Then it becomes clearer what step to take next for health and healing.

6. Take walks and mental and physical breaks to tune-up the connections. If you are concerned about dysfunction through disuse, then don't shun the activities. Find methods and opportunities to use your skills.
7. Appreciate that your mental recollection and physical movement are mutually dependent on each other, so work to preserve both activities with a passion to connect and benefit all.
8. There may come a time when you can no longer physically do and achieve certain acts. When this happens, let the ego go! If you cannot physically do or show, accept the change and move forward to think through how the message or instruction can be conveyed in an effective descriptive manner.
9. When you are an openly physical person, it is life transforming to no longer have the same ability and strength to command your body; or lost due to MS. Rather than crawl in a corner and vanish into nonexistence, learn to see your story as a positive example to motivate action and inspire greatness in others dealing with their situation. A true and forthright story can make a difference to someone living with a disease, giving specific hope to the present and vision for the next day.

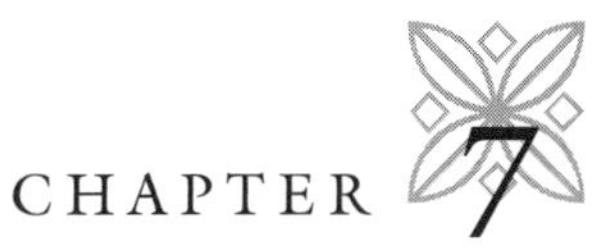

CHAPTER 7

Recognizing Cognitive Problems that Occur in Multiple Sclerosis: Defining the Cause

Patricia Kennedy, RN, CNP, MSCN

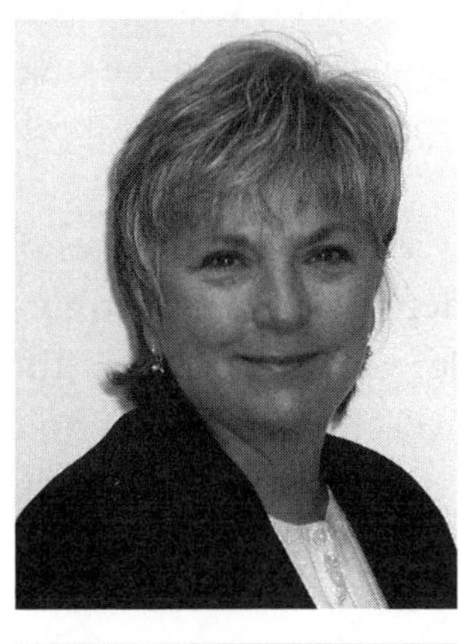

Pat Kennedy is a nurse practitioner whose clinical practice is with patients with multiple sclerosis only in Englewood, Colorado. She is the nurse educator for The Heuga Center in Edwards, Colorado, and nurse educator for the Rocky Mountain MS Center in Englewood, Colorado.

As few as 20 years ago, people diagnosed with multiple sclerosis (MS) were told "MS affects physical function, but your mind will be spared." This kind of news was certainly reassuring to individuals with newly diagnosed MS. Unfortunately, it was not always true, and people began to wonder why they were having trouble at work, at home, and at play doing tasks that used to come easily to them.

In the 1980s, information was gathered that showed, in fact, that cognition could be affected in MS. This opened our minds to the potential of improving how we can manage that segment of MS and its effects on people with MS, their families, and their participation in society.

As most people with MS will tell you, however, nothing is simple or straightforward. Other factors can cause or complicate problems with cognition. Other culprits can be mood issues, such as depression and anxiety, and fatigue. It is very difficult, sometimes, to differentiate between these factors to clearly identify the cause of cognitive dysfunction.

If you don't have problems with your thinking skills, never have had, or never will have, then this chapter may have less meaning for you. There is a rare person among us, however, who at some time or another does not experience issues related to being so tired you "can't think straight," being under so much stress that you can't remember common information, or being so depressed (or grieving or anxious) that planning ahead or doing simple tasks seems too difficult.

People with MS may experience these problems as well, but, because of their disease, other problems may occur, such as keeping up the pace at home or work or struggling with multitasking, keeping track of daily appointments, starting and finishing projects, and following conversations.

Our purpose in this chapter is to describe the similarities of cognitive dysfunction caused by MS, depression, and fatigue. Knowing these differences may guide you to manage the symptoms differently. Sometimes, however, we don't know what is causing the problem, so we do our best with the tools we have.

Cognition: What Is It?

Cognition is our brain's ability to think. Thinking involves many aspects, including our culture, abilities, experiences, education, insight, and logic. Other tasks involved in cognition and that may be affected by MS include the ability to

- Understand language and express ourselves
- Concentrate, shift attention, and multitask
- Learn and remember new information
- Plan and perform complex tasks
- Solve problems

In MS, it is estimated that 45% to 75% of people have some cognitive dysfunction in one or more of these areas.[1] Usually, it is mild. It is not related to physical disability and it may occur early in the disease. Sometimes, it is the first symptom that people experience. There are some people who only experience cognitive dysfunction and no other MS symptoms.

Cognitive dysfunction seems to be most closely correlated with increased numbers of lesions in the brain in general and with involvement of the corpus callosum.[2] The corpus callosum is a collection of fibers that allow the right and left sections of your brain to communicate, which is important to accomplish complex tasks. Cognitive dysfunction is also found when there is increased atrophy (tissue loss due to lesions) of the brain.

Studies have been done to determine if findings on magnetic resonance imaging studies can directly correlate to neuropsychological testing. The total number of lesions in the brain seems to be more related to problems with recent memory and abstract or conceptual reasoning. Lesions in the corpus callosum are more related to problems with the speed of information processing, sustained attention, problem solving, and mental arithmetic.[3] MS-caused cognitive dysfunction affects the following domains.

Memory problems occur most frequently in 22% to 31% of people with cognitive problems. This can include memory of events and conversations and involvement of both learning and recall. Short-term memory is most affected and long-term memory is somewhat spared. It used to be thought that a person with MS and memory problems had the information stored but couldn't retrieve it. Now, however, it is felt that people with MS need more time and repetition to learn and store information but can retrieve it once stored.

Attention and information processing affects 22% to 25% of people with dysfunction. This means that there is a slowing of the speed of processing information and a slowing of mental functioning. People may have problems filtering out distractions and have problems focusing on more than one task at a time (multitasking).

Verbal fluency affects 22% of people with dysfunction. People describe problems with word retrieval and expression of words.

Executive function problems occur in 13% to 19% of people with dysfunction. These can present as difficulty with complex concepts as well as struggling to solve problems or make good judgments. Organization can be affected, making starting and completing projects more taxing.

Visual/spatial deficits occur in 12% to 19% of people with dysfunction. These include an impaired sense of direction and orientation in space. It may be more difficult to understand common objects and how they work, such as putting things together that are labeled as "easy to assemble."

Language is least affected, at 8% to 10%. When there are problems in this area, people cannot carry on a meaningful conversation. Conversing with someone else is more difficult because there is loss of ability to process the conversation and respond to it in an understanding way.

If dysfunction occurs, most people experience only one area affected (43% to 56%), but some may have multiple areas affected (20% to 22 %).

Signs and Symptoms of Cognitive Dysfunction

You or your family and friends might notice that you are having difficulty remembering or are having problems coming up with the word you want to say or forget thoughts midsentence. There might be a slowness in or inability to understand what is heard or written and in making decisions that make sense. Many people have trouble following directions and get lost in areas they know well. Performance reviews at work may not be as high as previously received, and it may take you much longer to do your usual job. Common daily tasks, such as balancing the check book, tinkering with the car, or baking a cake, may be harder. Automobile accidents may occur.

Diagnosis

The level of diagnostic evaluation depends on the purpose for the testing. Some people need to know how to live day to day with their problems and want practical strategies to use. Others may want to address continuing in the work place and need to know how to structure that. For people facing legal issues or applying for disability benefits, a full neuropsychological evaluation may need to be done to prove (or disprove) the presence of and extent of cognitive dysfunction.

Occupational therapists and speech language pathologists, especially those with increased knowledge and experience in this area, are helpful in determining what primary areas are affected and then working with people to teach compensatory cognitive strategies. They offer practical solutions to utilize at home and work, with the family, and in the community.

Neuropsychologists use many different tests to determine particular areas of the cognitive realm that are affected and then compare results of those tests against those of people without MS of similar age and education. This is a method that quantifies and qualifies dysfunction. The testing can also differentiate among mood disorders, dysfunction from MS, and dysfunction that might occur from some other physiologic or psychological source.

There are hundreds of individual tests used in this kind of evaluation and dozens more are developed each year.[3] Testing can take a few hours or many. There is no one set of tests used by all neuropsychologists. It is helpful to find a neuropsychologist who has tested many people with MS. Experience in the disease will help to narrow the field of tests, making it less taxing on the patient. A subcommittee of the Consortium of MS Centers has made a recommendation for a shorter cognitive screening battery, which is being utilized by many neurophysychologists.[4]

Generally speaking, the components of a neuropsychological test battery will include a test that measures the general fund of information of the individual and then will include one or many tests to look at attention/concentration, memory, language, visual/spatial functions, and abstract/conceptual reasoning. Testing should not require visual acuity, motor speed, or coordination for adequate performance because people with MS often are affected in these areas.[5]

Medications Commonly Prescribed in MS Can Cause Cognition Dysfunction

- Anticholinergics and antimuscarinics (bladder-control treatments)
- Antiepileptic drugs (used for seizures and pain)
- Anti-fatigue medications (control of fatigue)
- Benzodiazepines (used for spasticity, spasms, anxiety)
- Muscle relaxants (used for spasticity)
- Narcotics (used for pain)
- Tricyclic antidepressants (used for depression, sleep, bladder problems, and pain)
- Steroids (used for exacerbation treatment)

Medications That Might Help Cognitive Dysfunction

There are no medications available for cognition that have been approved by the Federal Drug Administration for use in MS. You might discuss with your neurologist the possibility of using medications developed for use in other diseases with cognitive dysfunction, such as Aricept (donepezil), Namenda (memantine), and Provigil (modafinil).

Fatigue

Fatigue occurs in 75% or more of people with MS. It can limit activity more than any other symptom and is frequently the most disabling symptom of the disease.[6]

Definitions

1. A feeling of physical tiredness of lack of energy that many people experience (general fatigue).
2. A subjective lack of physical or mental energy, or both, that is perceived by the individual or care partner, or both, to interfere with usual and desired activities (MS fatigue).

MS fatigue comes on easily, without warning, and prevents sustained physical activity. Heat worsens this. It appears early in the disease and is not related to the amount of disability a person might have *and may affect both motor and cognitive dysfunction.*

Signs and Symptoms of MS Fatigue

People with MS fatigue experience a physical tiredness more quickly doing usual activities but can also experience a mental tiredness doing activities requiring more thinking or concentration, which we call "brain fatigue." When fatigue is a factor, it is harder to get motivated to do activities, just as it is harder to do activities that require concentration, such as reading or computer work. Fatigue at work may decrease your ability to perform up to your potential. You can see how these symptoms are similar to the ones seen in cognitive dysfunction due to MS lesions.

Other signs and symptoms of MS fatigue include feelings of depression, because of the fatigue and frustration of dealing with the fatigue, or anxiety, because activity and performance are now different and may be noticed by others. Although rest, sleep, or both may often lessen the fatigue, some people describe being tired all day. There is a fatigue that people experience called "short-circuiting fatigue." This occurs when a muscle group is asked to perform too long, such as when walking in the mall and needing to rest frequently. This also occurs when exercising but will resolve if rest is allowed.

Proposed Theory as to the Cause of MS Fatigue

The actual cause of MS fatigue is not clear but is felt to be a combination of immune system irregularities, central nervous system damage, and heat that affects conduction of messages related to physical activity.

It is important to not assume that all fatigue in MS is related to the disease. All other potential causes need to be considered. If there are other causes, they need to be treated first. If there are no other causes or if management of the other problems does not improve the fatigue, then it could be assumed to be true MS fatigue.

Another cause of fatigue might include sleep deprivation due to abnormal bladder function, breathing problems, leg movement, and pain. Deconditioning due to lack of exercise over time or poor nutrition will contribute to fatigue. When people incur some disability, such as weakness or spasticity, it consumes more energy to do activities. Some of the medications used in MS symptom management, such as baclofen, clonazepam, tizanidine, and gabapentin, can cause fatigue.

People with MS are not exempt from developing other health problems such as thyroid disease, anemia, cardiovascular disease, kidney and liver disease, and cancer. So when fatigue occurs, the work-up must be complete. Finally, depression and anxiety can cause fatigue.

Depression

Depression is defined as a syndrome of signs and symptoms that are episodic or clustered and are both psychological and physiologic. It is estimated that 17% of the general population experience a major depressive episode in their lifetime. In MS, the incidence is higher at 60% or greater.[7] This is a higher percentage than is seen in other chronic disabling diseases, which suggests more than a reactive response to a disease. It is believed that there is a physical change related to demyelination in the brain with MS that leads to depression. People with a purely spinal-cord form of the disease are less likely to have depression. There is some evidence of an increased risk of developing depression in patients who have increasing brain atrophy.

Signs and symptoms of depression include

- Feelings of sadness or despair
- Loss of interest in or enjoyment of activities
- Fatigue and sleep disturbances
- Appetite changes
- Inability to concentrate
- Psychomotor slowing (slowed movements and thinking)
- Irritability or anxiety

People with MS may experience increased symptoms of depression when the disease is newly diagnosed, when they experience a change in or loss of physical function, when there is decreased social support, and when MS is diagnosed at a younger age. The incidence of depression in men and women is similar.

Diagnosis

Depression is under recognized and under treated, in general, but especially in people with MS. Sometimes this comes from lack of communication about symptoms of depression with the healthcare provider. Culturally, admitting depression can be difficult for some. For others, recognizing depression is difficult because it may not present "classically" with the symptoms mentioned above. In the healthcare provider's office, lack of time and inhibition of communication about the topic may limit awareness on both sides.

Even if a person has some of the symptoms of depression but the symptoms are not overwhelming, treatment of those symptoms with antidepressants generally helps and improves quality of life. Depression is not a personal failure. Many people without MS are depressed. Treating depression is not difficult. Admitting to having depression seems to be difficult.

As in the case of fatigue, it is important to note how many of the signs and symptoms of depression are similar to those seen in cognitive dysfunction due to MS.

Management of Cognitive Dysfunction

If you experience cognitive problems and you have MS, you now know that the cause can be multifactorial. Having discussions with your healthcare provider about your symptoms will help determine the cause and will guide treatment. It is not always clear, however. There may be some trial and error before you find the management that works best for you. Please don't give up if the first attempt is not successful.

Cognitive Dysfunction Due to MS

There are many ways to compensate for whatever cognitive dysfunction you might experience. Be creative and do what works for you. Be flexible. Some tasks you can figure out on your own. If you have problems, however, seek advice from an occupational or speech therapist. Involve your family in your endeavors by sharing frustrations with finding coping strategies. Share your successes, too. The following sections include suggestions for both people with MS and their families.

Memory

Keep your mind stimulated by choosing activities that are simple and can give you the gratification of success. Starting off with the *New York Times* crossword puzzle when you've never done one before might set you up for failure. Some other examples of mind stimulators include word-search games, card games, TV game shows, and reading or listening to books on tape. If concentration is a problem, pick shorter books or limit reading to a chapter. Remind yourself of scheduled times by using a kitchen timer or wristwatch with an alarm. When away from home, call your answering machine to leave yourself messages, or try using a small recording device to capture your thoughts.

Plan for your medical appointments by listing your top concerns in writing and prioritize them. Bring a list of medications, times taken, and dosages to the healthcare provider for her to keep. Be sure to include over-the-counter treatments and supplements in the list.

Family Intervention

It is recommended that a family member also attends medical appointments to keep notes, ask questions, and provide information that may be forgotten. Family members can help organize medications, if appropriate, and provide reminders to take them, if needed. Most importantly, remember that memory loss is not willful.

Attention/Speed of Processing

If people are speaking too fast for you, then ask them to repeat the information for you or to slow down their speech. When on the phone, if you find yourself distracted or fatigued, ask the caller to call back to leave a message on your voicemail that you can retrieve later. You can also deal with distractions by going to another room or a quiet corner to hold conversations or by turning off the radio and TV while trying to do other tasks. Speaking on your cell phone while driving is dangerous (whether you have MS or not)! Do one task at a time before moving on to another because, once you leave a task, it takes much more effort to come back to it and pick up where you left off. Stay alert! If fatigued, step away for a short while to rest and retry later.

Family Intervention

Family members need to remember to speak more slowly and give information one part at a time to avoid overwhelming the person with MS. Repeat the information if needed, and ask for confirmation of understanding by having them repeat it back to you. Eliminate distractions when possible.

Verbal Fluency

If you have "tip of the tongue" problems—relax. The words will come or you can describe the word in a different way.

Family Intervention

Try not to show frustration or try to be helpful by redirecting the conversation. It is appropriate to assist only after trials have failed.

Executive Function

There are many types of organizational aides to help you. You could use pill boxes for medications; day planners, date books, or calendars for your schedule; and a family calendar to keep track of all activities in a single location. Some people like to use electronic organizers or tape recorders, whereas making a "to do" list is a good idea as long as it is consistently kept in one place. The list should be prioritized and realistic, breaking everything into steps, and should take into account the time needed to accomplish the tasks.

Writing everything down when you have a thought or information is helpful, but "yellow stickies" all over the house is not. Keep the notes all together. Sort through mail when it comes, keeping only what is important and tossing out the junk. Sort bills for payment, and organize a system that reminds you to do that. If you are the bill payer, have someone check your work. Make major decisions carefully...write out pros and cons...run it by someone else before instituting (if possible).

Family Intervention

If you are helping in this area, plan attainable goals, avoid unrealistic expectations, and recognize and allow successes. All family members should make their own entries on the family calendar and make sure everyone else in the family is aware of these entries. In decision-making situations, be loving and sensitive when guiding best decisions.

Visual/Spatial Information

Keep maps and important phone numbers in your car and get a GPS if possible. If you continue to have problems with driving, such as accidents, getting lost, and realizing the family won't drive with you any more, then seek out a driving evaluator (usually a specially trained occupational therapist found at rehabilitation centers) to test your driving. Often, they can make suggestions to make driving safer and easier for you. They might suggest that you not drive. That may be scary for you, but, if it keeps you from injuring yourself or someone else while driving, it would be better.

Family Intervention

If driving is an issue at your house, ask the healthcare provider to intervene.

Cognitive Dysfunction Due to Fatigue

Treat any underlying problems first and do all tasks in the time of day when you have the most energy. If your job or home responsibilities require that you spend long periods "thinking" (planning, organizing, computer work), then take mental vacations each hour when you let your mind go away to someplace stress free. When refreshed, come back to the original task before starting another one.

An occupational therapist can teach you fatigue-management skills and energy-conservation techniques. The best advice is to REST!! Sometimes just a few minutes of rest or sleep is enough to recharge your mental capabilities. Ask your healthcare provider for a prescription for REST, and paste it someplace conspicuous for you and your family to see. The other best advice is to exercise! Exercise, especially aerobic, will increase endurance and improve fatigue. It would be ideal to start with a physical therapist who understands neurologic diseases like MS. A physical therapist can evaluate your strengths and weaknesses and design an exercise program that is safe and appropriate.

Fatigue might interfere with your ability to think clearly. Delay important decisions or do less mentally challenging tasks until rested. Let your family and friends know when your energy is low. They aren't mind readers. Communication between family members is one of the best tools you can use to help everyone in the family function better.

Medications to Help Improve Fatigue

Although there are no medications approved by the Food and Drug Administration for use in MS for fatigue management, a discussion of fatigue symptoms with your healthcare provider might prompt him to suggest a medication, such as amantadine, Provigil (modafinil), or others. to be used off label.

On the alternative side, many people with MS use caffeine to help deal with their fatigue. A word of caution would be that caffeine works quickly, but the benefit also decreases quickly, leaving a person sometimes more tired than before. If you have bladder problems as part of MS, the use of caffeine is discouraged.

Dysfunction Due to Mood Issues

Please know that mood issues can be treated. If you feel you may be depressed, discuss it with your healthcare provider. If you feel "blue" but not depressed, still discuss it with you provider. Treatment for both issues includes a dual approach of medications and psychotherapy for best results. Treatment will improve symptoms (if related to mood) and improve quality of life. Psychotherapy is helpful at any stage on the continuum of MS. You will experience many changes over your life, and, although most are mild and manageable, some are not. Speaking with a psychotherapist will help you through those rough spots.

Psychotherapists can be licensed clinical social workers, psychiatric nurses, or psychologists. It would be important to ask your healthcare provider for recommendations. Not all therapists are licensed or appropriate. Talk therapy varies depending on the therapist you see. Discuss your needs and expectations, and, if you don't feel comfortable with the proposed plan, then find another therapist. One size does not fit all. Utilizing an antidepressant while you do talk therapy may help you manage your mood better while you are working through the issues.

Relationships and Cognitive Dysfunction

Cognitive dysfunction touches everyone involved with the person who has it. In fact, they are frequently the ones who detect changes first. It is awkward to discuss these issues with someone who seems unaware or doesn't want to admit there is a problem. Increasing evidence of decline in cognition and decreasing communication about it causes rifts in relationships, on the job, and with other responsibilities. It is important to open discussions with all people involved.

At home: Your family members should be made aware of the problems. Awareness may explain many observed behaviors and helps to "clear the air" and will lead to better understanding and communication.

At the physician's office: Many visits are short, and subtle changes may not be noted. It helps when family members share their observations with the healthcare provider prior to the appointment or at the appointment.

At work: If your employer and coworkers are aware of your cognitive problems, then sometimes accommodations can be made. However, if you have not told them of your diagnosis or issues you are having, no accommodations can be made. You cannot rely on protection from the Americans with Disabilities Act if you have not informed your employer of your disability. When employers are not aware of your MS or any cognitive dysfunction as a symptom of MS, they may terminate you based on poor performance. However, if you feel you are managing your job and its requirements well, you DO NOT have to inform your employer of your MS. In reality, though, cognitive changes are frequently the reason people apply for disability insurance.

Community responsibilities: Family members and other support-system members may need to guide someone with deficits to other activities or out of activities altogether. Overcommitting causes problems for most of us anyway, but, to the person with cognitive dysfunction, it can be overwhelming.

Moving Forward

Cognitive dysfunction is a sneaky adversary. For most, its onset is subtle until, one day, you realize that something you used to consider quite "doable" is suddenly not. The good news is that many problems it causes are manageable. For most people, the problems are mild and the management reasonably easy. For others, more family involvement may be necessary to make it all work. In all cases, having a good, open relationship with your healthcare provider is crucial so you can all work as a team.

Awareness of the potential causes of cognitive dysfunction may be enough to help you make compensatory changes. Knowing that fatigue and mood play major roles and blur the lines may make management more difficult. Educating your friends and family will help all of you, and your friends and family members can assist you with your strategies.

Conclusion

Being aware that there are several symptoms commonly seen in MS that may alter cognitive function, such as fatigue, mood changes, and MS lesions, will help you find the treatment and strategies appropriate to the cause. Communicating openly about these problems with family and friends will allow them to assist you in your efforts.

Be kind to yourself. "Misery comes free. Joy, fun, and laughter take planning."[8]

Mental Sharpening Stones and Perspectives

1. People with MS need more time and repetition to learn and store information but can retrieve it once stored.
2. In MS, it is important not to assume that all symptoms are caused by the disease. All other potential causes need to be considered. This applies to cognitive dysfunction, fatigue, and depression.
3. Your healthcare provider is the best person to help you delineate what is causing your cognitive dysfunction. Because the dysfunction could be related to MS lesions, MS fatigue, or depression, you need someone to help tease out the cause of your symptoms.
4. A "one-size strategy" does not fit all. Keep trying until you find the strategies that work best for you and your family.

References

1. Rao SM, Leo GJ, Bernardin L, Unverzagt F. Cognitive dysfunction in multiple sclerosis; frequency, patterns and prediction. *Neurology* 1991;41:685–691.

2. Rao,SM. Cognitive function in patients with multiple sclerosis: impairment and treatment. *Int J MS Care* 2004;Spring:9–22.

3. Lezak MD. Principles of neuropsychological assessment. In: *Behavioral Neurology and Neuropsychology.* Feinberg T, Farah M, eds. New York: McGraw-Hill; 1997:43–54.

4. Benedict RH, Fisher JS, Archibald, CJ, et al. Minimal neuropsychological assessment of MS patients: a consensus approach. *Clin Neuropsychol* 2002;16:381–397.

5. Peyser JM, Rao SM, LaRocca, NG, Kaplan E. Guidelines for neuropsychological research in multiple sclerosis. *Arch Neurol* 1990;47(1):94–97.

6. Krupp LB, Alvarez LA, La Rocca NG, Scheinberg, L. Clinical characteristics of fatigue in multiple sclerosis. *Arch Neurol* 1988;45: 435–437.

7. Minden, SL, Schiffer, RB. Affective disorders in multiple sclerosis. Review and recommendations for clinical research. *Arch Neurol* 1990:47:98–104

8. Metcalf, CW. *Lighten Up*. Reading, MA: Addison-Wesley; 1993.

CHAPTER 8

Time Out

Shelley Peterman Schwarz

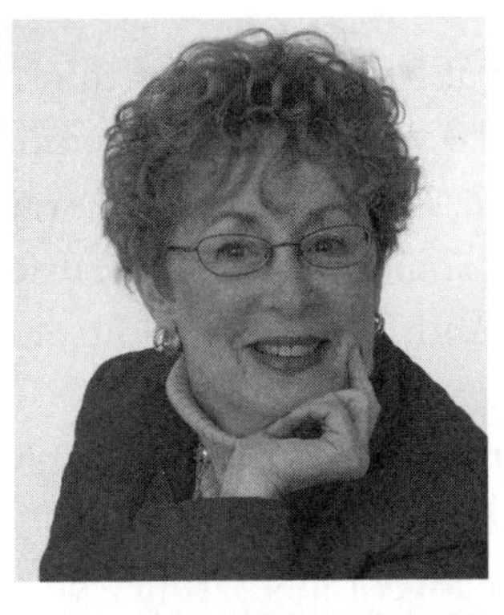

Author Shelley Peterman Schwarz writes the national syndicated Tips for Making Life Easier™ column and hosts the weekly Making Life Easier Internet radio program where she shares strategies and personal stories for living with multiple sclerosis.

When I was diagnosed with multiple sclerosis (MS) in 1979, I was told that MS did not affect cognition or a person's ability to think. I liked that answer, and for several years I had no reason to question it. Then I participated in some experimental MS treatments.

The first was in 1982, when I underwent hyperbaric oxygen treatments. One of the participants, "Mr. X," also had MS. Since we were together every morning, five days a week for a month, I tried to engage the man in conversation. All my efforts failed. His wife and my mother visited in the waiting room for the three hours that "X" and I were in the hyperbaric chamber. My mother learned and later shared with me the kinds of "thinking" problems this man was having at home. I thought it odd but rationalized it. Perhaps this man had another diagnosis in addition to MS.

The hyperbaric oxygen did nothing to slow the daily physical deterioration I was experiencing. So, a few months later when I qualified for a National Institutes of Health (NIH) double-blind study using chemotherapy and plasmapheresis to slow the progression of a MS, I "jumped" at the chance. It was during my three-week hospital stay for this study that I met people who told me that they felt they were having problems with their short-term memory, word-finding abilities, and "mushy-headed" thinking. Since I didn't think I was having any problems in these areas, I brushed off that information.

A few years after the NIH study, the National MS Society reported that 42% to 65% of the people who have MS experience cognitive problems. That got my attention! I started thinking about what that meant for me.

My doctor assured me that I'd know if I had problems thinking, and, if I didn't have them by now, (10 years after my diagnosis), I never would have them. It was true. I've never lost my way in my neighborhood. I've never lost my ability to time a meal so everything comes out at the same time. And, I've never had trouble following a complex set of directions.

However, as I look back, I realize that the reason I probably haven't noticed as many cognitive problems as I might have is because I compensate. In fact, I've been compensating every day for years. I hope some of the strategies I've used to compensate, and the solutions I've discovered, will validate your experiences and give you new ideas for coping with your cognitive challenges.

The most recent example of how I cope with cognitive-related issues happened as I was writing this chapter. I wrote a rough draft and sent it to Jeffrey Gingold, the author of *Facing the Cognitive Challenges of MS* and this book, *Mental Sharpening Stones: Managing the Cognitive Challenges of Multiple Sclerosis.* I wanted Jeffrey's feedback. We agreed to talk by telephone, and I explained that I'd like to record our conversation using the equipment I use to record my Making Life Easier™ Internet radio program, (which you can find at www.MakingLifeEasier.com)

After our conversation, I began to make the editing changes to my rough draft. I was working on several writing projects at the same time, and, in the course of saving one of the projects, I accidentally saved it over the newly edited chapter I was working on.

I didn't realize my error until about 10 days later when I went to finish up my editing. I was shocked, speechless, and sick to my stomach when I realized that the rough draft with the changes was gone!

I diligently back up my work every day, using a portable hard drive, a flash drive, and CDs. I also have MS Word make an automatic backup copy of every file. You could say I'm a little paranoid; however, in the 20 plus years that I've been using a computer, I've learned one can never have too many backups, especially if one has any cognitive challenges. Then it's really best to back up early and often.

Unfortunately, when I backed up the book chapter, it overwrote the previous version, and I lost all the changes I had made. I was not a happy camper because I was very close to finishing the assignment and HOW EMBARRASSING! As a professional writer, missing a deadline, making excuses, or not following through on agreements is a death knell for your career. You don't get a second chance. I would have been beside myself if the writing project wasn't about cognitive issues.

It was agonizing to admit to Jeffrey that my chapter would take a little longer than I thought. Thankfully, I still had the audio recording of Jeffrey's feedback, and he generously offered his written notes to supplement the audio file. And, thankfully, he was kind and understanding. We ended up commiserating and comparing other cognitive, professional horror stories.

In the end, I tried to take comfort in the fact that everyone has problems with their computers from time to time, and I was no different. And I waxed philosophical. No one was bleeding.

No one was in pain and, in three weeks, what difference would it make? So, it would take me a little extra time to rewrite my words. In the great scheme of things, this was not a life or death issue.

Even with the aggravation that computers can create, I use mine every day for gathering information, entertainment, staying connected, and working. The computer also helps me compensate for some of my cognitive problems, like forgetting how to spell common words, searching for keywords to see if I wrote about something before, and taking copious notes of telephone conversations so I can remind myself of past conversations, (just to name a few). I use a voice-activated, computer software program called, Dragon NaturallySpeaking—version 9.

I remember the first time I saw voice-activated software. It was at an Abilities Expo in Chicago where vendors showcase independent and assisted-living products and services helpful to people with disabilities. (These annual tradeshows are held in major cities across the country. Visit www.AbilitiesExpo.com to learn where to find the nearest Abilities Expo.) I loved the idea of voice-activated software, but, at the time (1980s), the program was $16,000. A little too hefty for my budget.

Fast forward to 2007; voice-activated software has become much more affordable. For less than $200, you can purchase an excellent and amazingly accurate voice-activated program that's compatible with all the major computer programs like Word, Outlook, Internet Explorer, Excel, PowerPoint, QuickBooks, ACT!, and others.

As my interest in writing increased and my hand strength and mobility decreased, I had to look for ways to make writing easier. About 10 years ago, I bought my first version of Dragon NaturallySpeaking (Nuance) software, which includes a microphone headset, and I have been using the program ever since. It's VERY SIMPLE to install.

The only drawback is that if you forget that you're wearing the microphone headset and drive away in your wheelchair, you'll pull out the wires and ruin the headset. (That would be me!) When that happens, you need to purchase a new microphone headset (about $20) and retrain your voice files with the new mike. Note: You also have to retrain your voice files when you purchase a program upgrade and decide to use the new microphone headset that comes with every program.

As a one-handed typist, I can talk much faster than I can type, so using voice-activated software makes me much more productive. A spellchecker corrects my spelling so I don't have to remember complicated or troublesome words. A personal idiosyncrasy that I deal with is that I'm reluctant to use Dragon when other people are around. I get tongue tied and self-conscious. It's not that I'm saying anything I shouldn't be saying. It's that it takes me a very long time to compose my thoughts, and I do a lot of writing and rewriting. I don't want others to know how I struggle.

The issue is that, because I'm so disabled, I'm rarely alone. During the day, while my husband, Dave, is away in his office at work, I'm in my home office running my business, Meeting Life's Challenges, LLC. Every day one of the company's employees is working in the same room with me. We each have our own jobs and areas of responsibility. However, my coworker can hear everything I say. Most of the time, I save my real writing time for nights and weekends when I'm alone in the office and Dave is busy doing things in other parts of the house. Then, no one can see or hear how slowly my mind works or how convoluted my thinking can be.

When I'm concentrating and the words are not coming, I have to talk out loud, starting and stopping, rephrasing, repeating phrases over and over again, until I find the right words with the right meaning. It can be an agonizing process, especially on days when I'm not well-rested, coming down with something, or stressed out by my MS-related limitations.

What would I do if I didn't have this kind of technology to make my life easier? I suppose I'd be a better "hunt and peck," one-handed typist. I know I would miss the funny things the program thinks I have said, like the time I was dictating tasks on my to-do list and I said, "Make an appointment with the gynecologist for a Pap smear." It came out on the computer screen "Make an appointment with the Gyna Colleges and Pabst beer." Or, the time I was dictating the notes I'd taken at a National Multiple Sclerosis Society fundraising meeting. I said, "Ideas for how we might go about filling up the tables at the luncheon." It came out, "Ideas for how we might go about killing off the tables at the luncheon."

For my most recent flub, I said, "My daughter is due 3 months after my daughter-in-law." And it came out, "My daughter is due 23 months after my daughter-in-law." (I don't think my daughter would have found it nearly as funny as I did.)

The other thing I would miss about not having voice-activated software is that it keeps my brain from talking back to me while I'm trying to write. When I'm typing, my inner editor voice is constantly judging (mostly negatively) what I write: "That information isn't important. No one is ever going to read this. When your magazine editor sees this, she will wonder what you were thinking." However, when I'm using Dragon NaturallySpeaking, my inner editor disappears. My brain must be concentrating so hard that there's no room for negative voices.

Another technologic aid that I just discovered is my new 22-inch, widescreen monitor to use with my desktop computer. Even though I regularly increase the font size on my computer so that it's easier to see my work, there were many situations in which, when I did that, I couldn't see the whole page and had to scroll from side to side.

Having a large monitor has made a huge improvement in the amount of energy I use when I'm on the computer. I never would have believed that having a larger monitor would have made such a difference in improving my ability to focus and concentrate for longer periods of time. I'm also using better posture and not contorting my neck straining to see what's on the screen. It was well worth the purchase and it cost less than $200.

When I'm not using the computer, I write lots of paper notes because it gives me a better chance of remembering things. People know if they don't see me write it down, there's a good chance I'll need a reminder. When I'm with friends and want to write something down, like book recommendations, a recipe, an e-mail address, or the date of our next get-together, I give one of my friends my paper and ask her to write down the information. Nobody thinks twice about taking notes for me. Then, I don't have to concentrate on listening, writing, spelling, or getting the words or numbers in the correct order.

When I'm in social situations, like dinners with friends, parties, and family get-togethers, I find it more difficult to focus when there are side conversations, the TV is on in the background, or music is playing, especially if the music has words. I start to feel my anxiety level rising because I can't process the input fast enough and have to ask that things be repeated and explained so that I make certain that I understand what is said. Those are times that I give myself permission for a "time-out," mentally stepping away from the multiple inputs and allowing it to enter my brain at a more controlled or slower pace. When I mentally return from the "time-out," I am more connected and able to receive incoming information into my thoughts.

I write myself lots of reminder notes. If I don't have a piece of paper handy, I've been known to write a note directly on the palm of my hand. I leave nothing to chance—or my memory. Sometimes I ask people to send me an email with the information they want me to have. Since I'm unable to remember more than three numbers is a row, I keep a piece of paper and pencil by every phone so I can write numbers, names, dates, and times. To retrieve numbers on the answering machine, I play and replay, (and replay) the answering machine until I'm able to write down the whole sequence. Thank goodness for telephones with caller ID, redial, and speed-dial features. Those help, too.

I have learned to accept my weaknesses, some of which I had before my MS diagnosis. For example, from the time I was in elementary school, math has always been a struggle for me. My mother, brothers, husband, and two children excel in math, so it's very intimidating. I do think my already-weak math skills have gotten worse since MS entered my life. I don't "see" numbers in my head. They seem to float away and disappear. I struggle to do even the simplest computations in my head. Two-part processes, like adding numbers and then dividing them, stresses me to the point that my stomach gets queasy. However, I've learned to accept help.

Perhaps it's my age (61). I feel I've become more mature and accepting of my limitations. Really, in the great scheme of things, who cares that I'm slow in math? I've let go of my embarrassment. The teasing I get from my family makes even me laugh. I'm very comfortable telling people I need help figuring out the gas mileage, calculating the tip on a restaurant bill, or doubling a recipe. I'm not sure how much of my inability to do computations is MS and how much is just the way my mind has always worked. (I work hard not to blame everything on MS.)

Recently, a cognitively related experience and my reaction to it surprised even me. I was asked to join the board of directors of a local nonprofit. I had met a few of the board members over the years but did not know them well. At the first meeting, I was sharing my thoughts related to the discussion. My comments were clear and concise; I didn't struggle to find the right word or take too much time getting out my thoughts.

However, when I tried to follow-up on something one of the other people said, my mind went blank. I sat there speechless. I could feel my face begin to flush. Normally, feelings of embarrassment and humiliation would take over, but not today. Today it didn't rattle me. I simply smiled, said, "Oops! I lost my train of thought." And, in a funny, high-pitched voice, I added, "Never mind!" Everyone chuckled, including me.

From past experiences, I knew that as soon as I relaxed a little, the thought would return. If I panicked and started to think about how foolish and inadequate I looked in front of these very capable people, I'd sabotage my efforts to remember. So, when the thought came back, I wrote it down. (ALWAYS keep pen and paper handy.) The next time there was a break in the conversation, I raised my hand and with a huge smile on my face and a twinkle in my eye I said, "The errant thought has returned." Then, referring to my notes, I shared the information.

Was the situation embarrassing? Yes. Was I the only person in the room who had forgotten what they had wanted to say? No. Was I going to let the incident ruin the rest of the day? No. And I know that, the next time what I want to say leaves me speechless, I'll be much kinder to myself and not make it any bigger than it really is. I'll just get more practice using my funny, high-pitched, "Never mind."

Raising Kids

In those early parenting years, I often experienced times when my brain just couldn't handle any more. That's when the stress level in the whole house went up. Over the years, I developed a few stress-relieving strategies that made raising our children easier.

Our daughter Jamie was 5 and our son Andrew was 3 when I was diagnosed with MS. By the time they were in elementary school, I was exhausted by the end of the day because of all the noise, activity, and household responsibilities. My head felt so heavy I wanted to take it off and put it on the nightstand. The feeling reminded me what one of my hearing-impaired students blurted out one day to express his frustration: "Too much many!" Now I understand exactly what my student was feeling and my family knows the phrase very, very well.

I can't remember exactly when I made the rule that, after 9 p.m., I was off "Mommy duty." If the children wanted me to help them with their homework, a class project, or any activity requiring brain power, it had to be before then. After that, my brain was fried.

If you've ever experienced cognitive problems, you probably have gotten to the limits of your ability to put two thoughts together. That's what I mean when I say that my brain was fried. And this feeling doesn't always have to be related to having kids. Now that we're empty nesters, I still have times when it feels like my brain can't process any more input. Don't ask me what I want for dinner. Don't ask me what I did all day. Don't ask me who called or why. Not only do I have trouble recalling information, I also have trouble sequencing events and expressing my thoughts coherently. I feel like whining and crying, like a child who needs her thumb, special blanket, and a nap.

I was very grateful when I stumbled on a very powerful parenting strategy. The kids were arguing and I couldn't sort out who did what. My brain just couldn't handle the commotion and stress, so I sent both kids to their rooms. I told them they couldn't leave their rooms until they found a solution to their conflict and gave the other permission to come out. At first they shouted things like, "I'm never letting you out!" "I'm making you stay in your room for a million years!" It was interesting and eye opening to listen to them, knowing that I didn't have to get involved.

Within a matter of minutes, I heard the kids talking to each other and negotiating a peace. "I'll let you out if you let me out." It was an amazing moment for me and a strategy I used for years.

When the kids got older and their arguments were more complex and more heated, I didn't have the mental energy to get involved no matter what time of day it was. My response to problems like sharing the car, using the telephone, or scheduling time on the computer was "I'm not getting involved. You guys work it out." As I look back, I can see clearly how Jamie and Andrew learned to resolve conflicts and became excellent communicators. It's satisfying to know that maybe my cognitive limitations actually did have a positive influence in some areas of their lives.

My Career

Two years after my diagnosis, I had to give up my career as a teacher of the deaf because of my physical limitations. I went into a deep depression. I lost an important part of ME and my self-esteem plummeted. Who was I now that I wasn't a professional? Since I was so physically limited, having no use of my legs or my dominant right arm and hand and only minimal use of my left hand, I depended on a little Amigo®, a three-wheeled, battery-operated wheelchair to get around. I needed lots of help with everything, including getting dressed, using the restroom, making breakfast, driving, and more. If I was able to work, I'd need a full-time assistant to do everything from filing and stapling papers to carrying meeting materials and helping me in the restroom.

Realistically, I didn't have a wide selection of career options open to me. But, I thought, maybe I could write. Unfortunately, I'd never written anything more creative than, "Please excuse Jamie for being absent. She had a sore throat." So a career as a writer was a HUGE STRETCH. It took me many, many years and lots and lots of tears and frustration to unlock my talent and gain the confidence to say (and believe)—"I'm a writer."

When I thought about being a writer, I knew that I didn't have the mental stamina to go back to school. Taking tests and having deadlines for papers was more stress than I could handle. What I did do, however, was attend time-limited (one half day per week for three weeks) classes at a level that had no deadlines. I also took a note taker with me so I could just listen without worrying about taking down important information. Then, when I returned home, I could read the notes, process the information, and begin to put the knowledge to use. (In addition, my note taker could help me in the restroom.)

It's frustrating when you can't learn as fast as you used to and your brain reaches its saturation point way too quickly. I was unprepared for the negative thoughts that kept entering my mind, like, "I can't believe how long this is taking you to finish. A fourth grader could do a better job. Why are you wasting your time trying to climb this mountain?" Silencing those thoughts and taking baby steps forward was an everyday battle. I worked harder than I ever have before, saying (and trying to believe) positive messages like, "You can do this! Just start writing! Trust that the right words will come out. Just one more sentence."

Over the last 22 years, I've written seven books (three of them in 2nd editions) and published more than 500 articles and Tips for Making Life Easier™ columns, and I write regularly for numerous national, regional, state, and local magazines and Web sites. I feel like I'm a teacher again, only the subject matter is different, and that's helped me accept my limitations and feel better about myself. With all the challenges I've had to deal with, no one would have faulted me for slowing down, but I've learned that, by taking little steps every day, your efforts build and add to your self-worth. I still get sad, frustrated, and angry, but those feelings usually don't last long because I have positive, interesting, and meaningful activities in my life.

Being a Wife

Today, I'm much better at knowing my limits. And, even though my husband, Dave, and I no longer are dealing with the everyday stress of being parents, at the end of the day, my brain is still tired. I don't want to make one more decision, no matter how simplistic, like choosing a restaurant for dinner. "Just lower the lift on our wheelchair accessible van, turn off the radio, and drive," I tell him. After all these years, (38 years of marriage), my husband still doesn't quite understand what it feels like when your brain is tired of working even at minimal capacity. He just rolls his eyes and shakes his head and drives to his favorite restaurant!

Dave and I had been married for only 10 years when I was diagnosed with MS. He has always been a magnificent husband

and father, naturally stepping in and doing more as I lost abilities to do everyday tasks. I know I am incredibly lucky to have a husband like Dave. He is helpful in any way he can be. I just have to be honest with myself and tell him what I need.

I've been using an Amigo® for more than 20 years, so it's hard to forget that I have a disability. But I do believe Dave doesn't even see the scooter anymore…or the fact that I have a disability, for that matter. He never lets me use MS as an excuse for not going to social engagements, school activities, or neighborhood gatherings, and he's there to provide the needed assistance. I think the only issues that cause problems are the ones you can't see. Because he has always enjoyed excellent health, I think that Dave sometimes doesn't totally appreciate what it's like to have a chronic illness, especially one that includes cognitive problems.

When the kids were young, it was easy to understand the mental fatigue of raising children. However, now that the kids are out of the house, it's been a little harder to get him to understand why I need the radio turned off in the car, especially when we're trying to carry on a conversation. When there are too many things going on around me, I get anxious and agitated and lose energy like a balloon with a slow leak. I function better when there is only one thing to attend to at a time.

Dave is an amazing "multitasker," which is an almost nightly reminder of his abilities and a lack of mine. I admit it's frustrating when I just want to turn off the TV and read. He is comfortable simultaneously watching a TV program, reading the paper, and listening to a ball game through earphones!

He also needs a lot less sleep than I do. I need more quiet, less frenetic activity in my life. Dave can bounce from one thing to another, from early morning to late at night. Not me. That's why I disappear into my home office and "play quietly" on the computer. Dave doesn't understand how or why I spend so much time in my office. I explain it as being gentle on my brain. I can control the noise. I can control the volume. I can control the speed at which things move. I don't have anybody tapping their toes waiting for me. I can do something, read something, and listen to something over and over and over again, and no one knows it but me.

It's the nature of having cognitive difficulties. People who don't have them don't really understand what it means to have mushy-headed thinking, slowed abilities to receive and process information, or fatigue so great that one just can't think something through. I often wish there was some way to remind my family and friends of my cognitive deficits without becoming a pest or sounding like a broken record. Perhaps by reading my story, it will validate your experiences and help articulate to others what you'd like them to understand about "thinking problems."

Writing down some of my experiences has helped me give voice to things I've been feeling for a long time. It has been validating and comforting for me; I hope you find it the same.

Mental Sharpening Stones and Perspectives

Here are the concepts I feel help us cope with cognitive challenges.

1. Acknowledge that you have cognitive problems. (You can't change what you don't acknowledge.)
2. Know that you are not alone.
3. Give yourself the extra time you need to process and complete mentally taxing activities.
4. Give yourself a "time out" when you're overwhelmed, that is, a time and space where you can regroup and collect your thoughts.
5. Adjust, compromise, and accept help from people around you.
6. Tell people exactly what you need and how they can help you.

7. Everyone forgets. Don't blame everything on your illness.
8. Relax, the thought will return. (Then write it down.)
9. Accept who YOU are and try not to compare yourself to others.
10. Challenge yourself to find solutions to your problems.
11. Be open to new ideas, people, and experiences. Visit www.MakingLifeEasier.com for more tips, strategies, and encouragement.
12. Be kind, patient, and proud of yourself for solving problems big and small.
13. Share you tips and coping strategies with others.
14. Writing about your challenges (cognitive and otherwise) may be a way to release pent-up frustration and tension. Over time, that written record may also document how far you have come in accepting the new YOU.

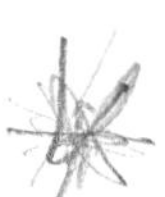

CHAPTER 9

Mind over Matter: Lessons in Problem Solving

Eynat Shevil, PhD, OTR

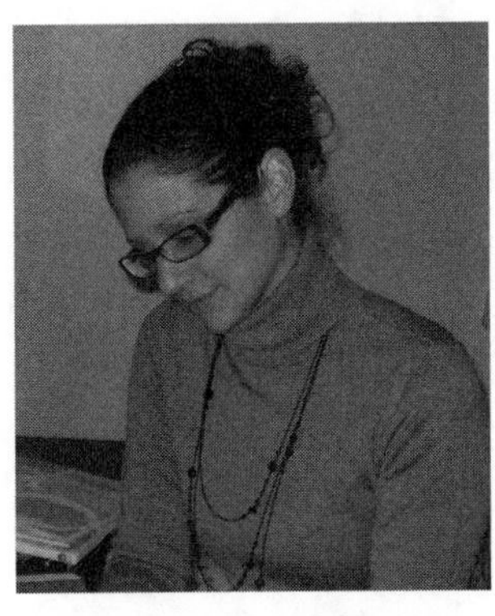

Eynat Shevil is an occupational therapist from Israel. She has recently completed a PhD in Disability Studies at the University of Illinois at Chicago. Dr. Shevil's research focuses on the impact of cognitive changes among persons with MS, as well as on developing intervention programs to manage cognitive challenges.

In a suburban hospital outside a metropolitan city, eight individuals with multiple sclerosis (MS) have gathered together to participate in a group-based education program. Both men and women are taking part; their ages range from 40 to 62. Some of them are full-time workers, whereas others have retired or are currently on disability. The majority of them are living with others: spouses, children, or other extended family members. Despite the diversity in the group, they all share at least one important characteristic: they are all experiencing cognitive changes as a result of MS. They have enrolled in a program called "Mind over Matter" to learn more about their cognitive changes and hopefully some ways to manage these symptoms' intrusive effect on their everyday lives.

For more than five years, I have been working with persons with MS, specifically on issues relating to cognitive symptoms and challenges. Through this work, I have identified a need for cognitive interventions that address the management of cognitive difficulties. For my doctoral research I developed and tested a group-based education program called "Mind over Matter: Learning to Manage Cognitive Symptoms in MS." The purpose of the program is to teach participants practical strategies to help manage cognitive challenges. The program was delivered in community settings and included five sessions that were conducted once a week.

During the program, participants gain insights regarding common cognitive changes that can occur in MS and their impact on daily activities, including changes in memory, difficulties with attention and concentration, slowed information processing, reduced visual-perceptual skills, and issues with executive functioning. A wide variety of strategies are demonstrated throughout the program, such as using lists and alarms to help remember, changing the surrounding environment or organizing spaces to make tasks easier, talking to yourself when confronted with particularly complicated tasks, and discussing cognitive changes with your doctor.

Increasing Your Knowledge about Cognitive Changes

When most people with MS are asked about their cognitive changes, they may give general descriptions such as, "I just can't focus," or "My memory is gone," or "I'm finding it hard to think straight." Although true, such statements do not give information on the nuanced impact of these changes. In addition, people don't know that many of the daily challenges they are experiencing are in fact cognitive changes. Rose* talked about this at the end of the program:

**All names have been replaced with pseudonyms.*

"Before I took the class I didn't understand why I was doing things the way I was doing them. I thought there was something wrong with me. I didn't understand why I was having all these difficulties. I didn't know what the root of it was. I didn't understand its connection with MS, so that has been very enlightening for me to have a better understanding. It reassured me knowing that it's from the MS and there are some resources that I can tackle it with."

If one is to tackle cognitive changes and find solutions to everyday problems, then you need to get specific. Many may not realize that the reason they sometimes blank out while driving may be due to problems processing visual information. Difficulties taking part in social engagements (for example, meeting with a group of friends for coffee) and following conversations are because the person's ability to process information may have slowed down. Difficulties figuring out complicated issues at work or at home can be the result of problems with executive functions (the higher mental functions of the brain that include solving problems, planning, reasoning, etc.).

Successful management of cognitive symptoms begins with educating oneself about the different changes that can occur in MS and how these changes can interfere with different daily activities that you want and need to do. These activities can include working, maintaining volunteer activities, being able to manage a household, engaging in leisure activities, taking care of family members, and socializing with others. It is important for people with MS to increase their knowledge regarding cognitive changes because this knowledge can increase their awareness of what is happening to them.

Betty, a school teacher, talked about how she didn't know that a lot of the problems she was experiencing were actually her cognitive changes. She was struggling trying to grade papers, having a hard time coming up with lesson plans, and trying to listen to more then one student at a time was becoming nearly impossible.

During the program, Betty learned that the difficulties she is experiencing are a result of her reduced ability to multitask (do more then one thing at a time) and slowed information processing. At the end of the program she commented:

"I'm more aware of my cognitive problems. I've increased my knowledge of cognitive changes and I can identify them."

For many of the participants, recognizing their problems and being able to give them a name was empowering and provided a heightened sense of control over this symptom. John, a retired banker said "[Learning about cognitive problems] helps you recognize and accept that it's a problem. It also shows you that there are things that you can do to help it."

Solving Cognitive Problems

Managing cognitive problems is more than just finding a solution to different problems as they arise. The final or appropriate solution is only the end product of a larger process that includes identifying the problem (at times easier said than done), learning what the problem is and what exactly it involves, brainstorming a variety of potential solutions that might work, and then picking out and trying the one solution you think is going to work best. This process is a problem-solving technique[1] that participants in "Mind over Matter" learn, and it is how they address every single cognitive problem that they encounter.

For example, at the beginning of the program, Jack identified his cognitive problem as difficulty with multitasking. In other words, when he tried to do more than one thing at a time, such as checking e-mails at work and talking on the phone, he got confused and distracted. Jack was encouraged to narrow this problem to a specific activity that he is finding difficult because problems with multitasking can happen during many activities, in which different solutions can apply. Difficulties with multitasking can happen at work and at home. However, the solution you apply at work may be very different than the one you apply at home, where you have more flexibility.

Jack reworked his problem and identified the following: I find it hard to do my daily household chores all at the same time (for example, doing laundry, dusting, sorting through the mail, and doing the dishes). I get distracted and I can't remember what I started. I end up forgetting things, like putting the laundry in the dryer, and I'm completely exhausted once I'm done. He then identified different strategies that he can use to make this activity easier. His options included delegating some of the chores to his children, considering hiring someone to clean the house, or spreading out chores throughout the week (such as doing one chore each day). Jack thought that spreading out the chores would work best for him. He tried it out and it worked!

By avoiding multitasking and doing one chore at a time, Jack was able to keep on task and maintain his responsibilities. Many participants found the problem-solving technique[1] beneficial for tackling cognitive problems. Sue summarized: "It made me sit down and think about problems. I'm better able to reason through it and think about it before doing it."

Using Strategies

Participants preferred to address cognitive problems and find solutions for them, rather than having to give up activities they needed and wanted to do. Experiencing cognitive problems can cause people to reduce the number of activities they participate in because the activities are too difficult or because they feel embarrassed. Some of the common activities that people drop are leisure activities (such as reading or going to the movies) and socializing. Learning to successfully manage cognitive problems can increase participation, as Helen commented: "I haven't given [activities] up but switched the way I was doing them because I have information to better manage instead of letting things go."

Rebecca loved playing bridge with her friends. However, as her cognitive abilities deteriorated, she found it increasingly more difficult to keep up with her game. She was getting confused between the different hands and couldn't keep the rules straight in her head. She slowly began to limit her bridge playing and finding reasons not to go. Rebecca didn't want to give up this enjoyable activity, and together the group brainstormed strategies that she can use to keep playing. Rebecca started to practice bridge at home using the computer. In addition, she wrote down the main rules of the game on small index cards that she took with her to bridge games. Her friends didn't mind that she periodically referred to these cards while they were playing. By incorporating these relatively simple strategies, Rebecca was able to continue playing bridge rather than having to give it up.

There is no single magic strategy that one can use to solve all cognitive problems. The "trick" is to figure out what strategies are going to work best for you, considering your specific roles and responsibilities and the tasks you find most challenging. When you find out what the best strategy is for you, then stick with it and see if you can apply it to other activities or situations that you encounter. Below are examples of solutions and strategies that participants in "Mind over Matter" began utilizing to tackle cognitive challenges.

Ruth began color-coding her schedule: "I use a calendar and a daily planner. Most important is written in red, medium in green, and least important in blue or black. I leave my planner on the table so I can see it."

James' favorite strategy was "multisensory input." If he wants to remember something, he has to "write it, see it, and say it out loud. The more input you get, the more cemented it gets."

Some participants found changing their environment particularly helpful to avoid confusion and help with their visual processing. Changing the environment included:

- Organizing spaces like desks, drawers, pantries, or closets using labeled compartment containers or baskets.
- Preventing clutter by throwing away or donating old magazines, unusable plastic food containers, clothes, etc.
- Always putting items back in the same place—keys, scissors, sunglasses, cell phone, etc.

Jill commented how this strategy helped her organize her kitchen: "It's so much easier to find what I'm looking for. It gives me confidence that I can generalize this to other areas of my life."

Other participants found it beneficial to incorporate routines and plan their activities throughout the day or week. Routines help keep you on track when your mind or focus tends to wonder. If you get distracted, you can go back to your activity list and pick up where you left off. You can plan cognitively demanding tasks during times when you are more alert and less fatigued. If you find yourself hitting a "cognitive wall," don't hesitate to postpone tasks that you had planned to a later time. For example, you may have planned an afternoon trip to the hardware store to purchase some gardening items. However, after spending the morning going through the mail and paying the bills, your mind is "foggy."

Ask yourself—Can the gardening tools wait? Do I have to get them today? What's the worst that can happen if I postpone this task to next week? Saving cognitive energy is very important, and you want to avoid complete mental exhaustion. Planning daily activities worked particularly well for David: "I know which part of the day I become tired. I plan more complicated things earlier in the day before I get tired. Less important things I plan for later or just don't do them."

Another popular strategy to help stay focused and improve memory is talking out loud and organizing your thinking before doing a cognitive task. Do you find yourself repeatedly having to return home after leaving to check if you turned off the stove or shut the garage door? If you accompany closing the garage door with saying it out loud (literally saying "I shut the garage door"), you are less likely to question if you did it. By saying something out loud, you are consolidating it in your memory and incorporating a level of consciousness that does not occur when you do things automatically or without thinking about them.

Organizing your thoughts before you start an activity helps prevent feeling scattered, especially for complicated tasks such as planning a family vacation. Before you sit down in front of the computer to research different travel options or pick up the phone to call your travel agent, take a moment to think through all the things you need to do to plan a successful vacation. You can even jot the steps in a notebook. Tracy commented how organizing her thoughts mentally prepares her: "[It] cuts away some of the chaos because you are more organized."

The Role of Stress

Reducing stress was discussed throughout the program. Many participants talked about how stress can make a lot of cognitively difficult tasks even more challenging to perform. Many people perform poorly or have difficulty concentrating when they are under stress, regardless of having a chronic disease. Stress related to cognitive symptoms can occur during tasks that are more difficult to perform (such as driving, balancing your checkbook, or figuring out what to pack for a business trip).

Stress can be further induced when attempts to complete the task are either unsuccessful or do not meet your standard of satisfaction. During the program, participants learned how stress can contribute to cognitive challenges and learned that simplifying activities and using strategies such as slowing down, completing one task at a time, and organizing their thoughts before taking on a cognitive task, can significantly reduce stress and improve cognitive abilities.

Linda is a corporate analyst. In general, she finds it difficult to concentrate at work because her role includes many responsibilities and her desk is located in a central location that sees a lot of "human traffic." Her biggest concern is facilitating business meetings when she has to attend to multiple people and keep track of what they are saying. This creates a significant amount of anxiety and stress for her: "At work I have a problem with focusing in large groups, so one of the strategies we came up with was for me to find out who the people were going to be at the meeting prior to the meeting and make a little column of their name, and then, once I'm in the meeting, I can just jot down what this person is saying and then write down what this person is saying. And then compile it later after the meeting. So then if I have questions, I can go back and look in there. So it just needs a little more tweaking for me but it was perfect."

Stress can be managed in a number of ways. Larry explained: "I can think easier without stress. I do so much better without it." Robert talked about how he does not beat himself up anymore if he is experiencing cognitive problems: "I'm kind of slowing myself down, taking time to rest more. It makes me more aware of what's going on." Finally, some participants reduced their stress by changing their view of cognitive problems. For example Barbara said: "I don't let [cognitive problems] bother me. I decided it's not worth it."

Changing Perceptions

Many people find it difficult to think positively or neutralize negative thoughts about cognitive changes. During "Mind over Matter," participants are given an exercise to complete. They are asked to write a negative thought or feeling they have about their cognitive changes and then try to reframe that thought into a more positive one. Some participants modified their negative perceptions by stating that they now have the tools they need to manage their cognitive changes and can resume some of the valued activities they needed to give up. Some participants chose to focus on their successes rather than their challenges. Vera articulated this perspective: "You're sort of bred to think that you only deserve the carrot when you get the whole thing done. But now, in our situation, you deserve that pat on the back when you get the pieces done, the intermediate goals. That was really important to me because I'm really hard on myself."

Participants who had to quit their jobs, because cognitive difficulties were becoming too overwhelming, talked about how this transition was freeing up time to engage in other activities they would otherwise not be able to do.

One perception change made by Peter touched many members of the group. Peter was a full-time worker who spent many hours in the office. When cognitive changes set in, he was unable to continue working. Peter and his wife have three children. He transitioned, among other things, into the role of stay-home dad. During the perception exercise, Peter said that, although it was initially very difficult to quit working, spending more time at home is allowing him to see his children grow up and enjoy quality time with them. He perceives this transition as a gift and feels very fortunate to have this opportunity.

Gloria had many concerns and frustrations about her ability to find words while conducting conversations. She kept getting stuck and felt that she wasn't making any sense at all. Gloria started using some of the strategies she learned during the program to tackle word searching. She slowed down her speech, tried to conduct conversations where it was quiet so she could concentrate better, and, if she forgot a specific word, she would keep talking about the topic until the right word came out. She also told the people she was talking to that it was OK for them to "fill in" the word if they thought of it.

Using these strategies helped Gloria feel better and increased her confidence when talking to others. She still sometimes struggles finding the right words and gets stuck completing sentences, but her perception about this cognitive challenge has changed: "It's not like the problem really went away, but my reaction is different and it's very positive."

Sharing Cognitive Challenges with Others and Seeking Support

One of the most important things that participants learned in the program is the benefits of communicating cognitive changes to others, seeking support, and asking for help. A particularly powerful component of "Mind over Matter" was the group format in which the program was delivered. For some, it was the first time they talked about their cognitive challenges with others. Knowing that the other participants were going through similar experiences and frustrations created a safe environment for disclosure and sharing. Helen commented how she felt less alone in this endeavor: "Hearing others stories, sharing what other people have gone through, it let you know that you are not alone; that makes me feel better."

Sharing experiences, being able to relate to others, offering suggestions and ideas from personal experiences, and receiving positive reinforcement is extremely empowering. The group format allowed for discussions on different topics related to cognitive changes and fostered peer learning. For example, Tom mentioned that being able to brainstorm with the group gave him some solid ideas how to tackle his cognitive problems. Tom tends to get anxious in social gatherings when there are a lot of people around, and he loses his concentration and focus. He expressed this concern to the group.

Laura, who experiences a similar problem, offered a solution. Laura explained that, when she feels overwhelmed in group situations like parties, she takes a "time out" and goes to the restroom or steps outside where it's quiet. This "time out" helps her relax, calm down, and regroup. She can then return to the party with rejuvenated mental strengths. Tom said that the solution sounded reasonable and noted to try it himself. The following week, Tom happily reported to the group that Laura's suggestion was great and really helped him "stay grounded" when he met with a group of friends that weekend.

Cognitive changes are one of the hardest and most complex symptoms for others to understand and accept. This is because cognitive symptoms are invisible and impact not only the person with the symptoms, but the people around them as well. Your family may not understand why you forget errands that you said you would run, your friends may be concerned because you seem distant and pulling away, your supervisor may become aggravated that you are falling back on responsibilities at work, and your neighbor of 20 years may be hurt because you did not recognize her last week at the grocery store.

Although disclosure of cognitive changes can be complicated and at times not possible, there are many benefits to communicating cognitive changes with people *you feel comfortable with* (such as a close friend, your spouse, a trusted colleague at work, a volunteer at your local MS organization hotline). One can receive encouragement and support from others regarding cognitive difficulties. If you decide to share your cognitive difficulties with others, then consider accompanying that with a request for assistance. Assistance does not necessarily mean asking someone else to do a task for you. It can include help with brainstorming potential solutions, perfecting existing ones, holding you accountable, and making sure you are using the strategies. Together you can tackle cognitive changes as a team.

Jane has been struggling with cognitive changes for a few years now. Although her husband knew she was experiencing cognitive difficulties, he was unaware of the extent of these changes and how exactly they were impacting her ability to work. Jane gave her husband an information pamphlet about cognitive symptoms in MS, and, later, they sat down and talked about it. Jane's husband asked her many questions and found out things he did not know before about cognitive symptoms. She felt more comfortable talking about her difficulties at work and at home. Together they began talking about different strategies that Jane can use to lessen her stress at work and meet the demands of her job. Jane told the group that it was one of the best conversations she and her husband ever had about her MS, and it made her feel a lot better. She felt that she now had an ally in her efforts to manage cognitive changes.

On a Personal Note

Over the course of four months, I ran five "Mind over Matter" programs with a total of 35 participants. With each program, I had the privilege of witnessing a motivated, resilient, and self-sustaining group of individuals tackle cognitive changes and challenges head on. I was not the leader of the program, but, rather, my role was to *facilitate* the group process. I provided information on cognitive symptoms, demonstrated different cognitive solutions, and guided discussions. At the beginning of the program, it was my job to take more of a lead and guide a group of strangers through the process of managing cognitive symptoms. However, as the program went on, I found myself doing less and less of the talking. This was a natural result of the groups' development, one that I found particularly fulfilling.

Participants felt comfortable raising cognitively challenging tasks, whereas other members spontaneously chimed in offering valuable feedback, practical suggestions, and advice about how to solve the problem. During such exchanges, I could sit back and reflect on the dynamic that presented itself before me. The participants were indeed the experts on their lives and unique circumstances and were learning how to independently overcome difficulties. This mutual exchange of support was beneficial for both the givers and the receivers, and I felt confident that this problem-solving process can continue after the program ends.

※ Recommendations for Managing Cognitive Changes

- *Educate* yourself about the common forms of cognitive changes that can occur in MS and how these changes can interfere with your ability to do everyday activities. It is also important to understand how these changes interact with other MS symptoms.
- *Talk to your healthcare provider* (physician, neurologist, nurse practitioner) about your cognitive changes. Your provider can refer you to rehabilitation professionals, such as an occupational therapist, speech language pathologist, or neuropsychologist, for further cognitive evaluation and specific intervention.
- Never underestimate the power and benefits of *peer support.* Others like you can help brainstorm solutions and strategies to manage cognitive changes. Also, you can offer valuable support and ideas to others based on your unique life experiences. Seek peer support through MS support groups, on-line communities, or volunteer work at local or national MS organizations.
- Create situations that *work for you, not against* you. Think of ways to change your environment or the task that will increase the likelihood for success. Remember, there are many strategies for you to choose from. The key is finding the solution that works best for you. When you find that strategy, try to generalize it and apply it to other activities and see if it works.
- *Communicate* your cognitive changes to people in your everyday life with whom you feel comfortable sharing the information. They can help you find solutions to cognitive challenges and also hold you accountable to make sure you are sticking to your plan.
- You are far more likely to successfully engage in cognitively demanding tasks if you *reduce stress and fatigue.* Conserve

physical and mental energy. Avoid doing cognitively demanding tasks during times when you know you are tired or in environments that are loud or busy with activity.

- Avoid *multitasking*. Give yourself the mental space to process each task you want to do. You will be more efficient if you do only one task at a time and are able to complete it. Revisiting half-completed tasks wastes time and mental effort.
- Break big tasks into *smaller steps*—don't overwhelm yourself with a big project. Your goal is to maximize successes and minimize failures. Don't set goals or standards that you know are too high to achieve.
- *Think positively*. Although positive or neutral perceptions about cognitive changes are hard to consider, they can significantly contribute to your physical and mental well-being.
- *Healthcare professionals*—ask your clients with MS if they are experiencing cognitive changes because some people may be experiencing challenges without being aware of this symptom. Educate your clients about cognitive symptoms and their impact on daily activities. If needed, refer such clients for further cognitive evaluation and interventions. Provide written materials on cognitive symptoms that can be reviewed by the clients, their family members, or friends.

Acknowledgments

The information presented in this chapter originates from a research study conducted by Eynat Shevil at the University of Illinois at Chicago. The study was approved by the University Institutional Review Board (protocol number 2006-0477). Support for the research was provided by the American Occupational Therapy Foundation Dissertation Grant and the Deiss Endowment for Biomedical Research from the University of Illinois at Chicago. Dr. Shevil wishes to thank all the participants for sharing their experiences and generously providing valuable comments and insights.

Mental Sharpening Stones and Perspectives

This is a compiled list of compensatory cognitive strategies that you can select from and use to manage cognitive changes:

1. Before beginning a cognitive task, organize your thoughts and think through the steps you need to take.
2. Improve your cognitive performance by asking yourself questions as you are performing a task (for example, "Am I concentrating on my checkbook or is something else distracting me?").
3. Use mnemonics to help trigger your memory. Create a visual image in your mind to remember someone's name. Repeat tasks out loud as you are doing them—for example "I'm locking the front door."
4. Slow down, do one thing at a time, and avoid multitasking.
5. Think positively.
6. Make lists.
7. Use time-management sheets, a planner, or a calendar. Evenly spread out and prioritize cognitive tasks throughout the day or week. Color code your schedule.
8. Incorporate routines.
9. Don't engage in demanding cognitive tasks if you are stressed or fatigued.
10. Write down notes or use a dry erase board (at home or at work). Place notes where you are likely to see them.
11. Use flowcharts for complicated tasks that require multiple steps.
12. Perform cognitive tasks in cool or air-conditioned environments.

13. Organize spaces to prevent clutter. Keep items in the same place. Ask others who use the space to keep it tidy.
14. Do cognitive activities in a quiet area or during times when there are fewer people around. Turn off the radio and television (don't just turn down the volume).
15. When driving or visiting an unfamiliar location, study a map before your visit.
16. Use assistive technology, such as digital voice recorders, electronic organizers (personal digital assistant—PDA), alarms (e.g. watches, pill boxes with alarms), pagers, and cellular phones.

Recommended Readings

Consumer-based Books, Brochures, and Articles

Clear Thoughts on Cognitive Problems in Multiple Sclerosis. Published by: International Organization of MS Nurses (www.iomsn.org).

Gingold J, *Facing the Cognitive Challenges of Multiple Sclerosis.* New York: Demos; 2006.

LaRocca N, Kalb RC. *Multiple Sclerosis: Understanding the Cognitive Challenges.* New York: Demos; 2006.

LaRocca NG, King M. *Solving Cognitive Problems.* Published by the National Multiple Sclerosis Society (www.nmss.org).

Lou JQ, Tischenkel C, DeLange L. *Cognitive Deficits in Multiple Sclerosis.* Published by the Multiple Sclerosis Foundation (www.msfocus.org).

Myles R. Loosening the Knots of Cognitive Problems. InsideMS 2007. Published by the National Multiple Sclerosis Society (www.nmss.org).

Shi J, Khurana S. Cognitive Issues in Multiple Sclerosis. *Multiple Sclerosis Quarterly Report.* United Spinal Association (www.unitedspinal.org).

Turner DL. Notes from a [Former] Reader. *InsideMS 2004.* Published by: National Multiple Sclerosis Society (www.nmss.org).

Professional Journal Articles

Amato MP, Zipoli V, Portaccio E. Multiple sclerosis-related cognitive changes: a review of cross-sectional and longitudinal studies. *J Neurol Sci* 2006;245:41–46.

Brassington JC, Marsh NV. Neuropsychological aspects of multiple sclerosis. *Neuropsychol Rev* 1998;8:43–72.

Bobholz JA, Rao SM. Cognitive dysfunction in multiple sclerosis: a review of recent developments. *Curr Opin Neurol* 2003;16: 283–288.

Shevil E, Finlayson M. The experience of managing cognitive impairments among persons with multiple sclerosis. *Israeli J Occupat Therapy* 2006;15:E5–E22.

Shevil E, Finlayson M. Perceptions of persons with multiple sclerosis on cognitive changes and their impact on daily life. *Disabil Rehabil* 2006;28:779–788.

References

1. D'zurilla TJ, Nezu, AM. *Problem Solving Therapy: a Social Competence Approach to Clinical Intervention*, 2nd ed. New York: Springer Publishing; 1999.

CHAPTER 10

Advocating for True Fortune

Jeffrey N. Gingold

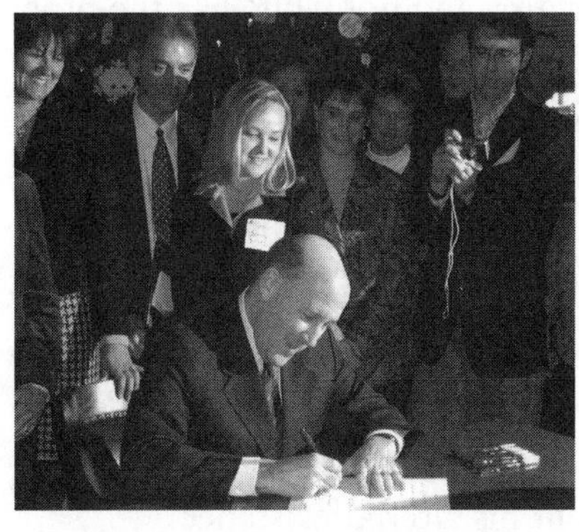

December 21, 2005 Governor Jim Doyle created a voluntary "check-off" on Wisconsin State Income Tax Returns for donations to fund MS programs.

"Difficult things we do quickly. The impossible takes a little longer."

David Ben-Gurion

"You have multiple sclerosis (MS)!" I would be reminded. "How can you feel fortunate?" they would ask. It may sound like an old Yiddish proverb, but I learned that my MS disability could be much worse—so I relish life, while pushing back against merciless exacerbations. Having a disease that is chronic and progressive is everything that it is cracked up to be, but that doesn't have to be an endpoint for a life.

Despite the sensation of walking, talking and thinking in an ocean of thickening molasses, I won't complain about where my life with MS had turned. It was a matter of clutching an honest perspective. Whether it was simple luck or good timing, my life would have been far crueler if I had been forced to deal with MS

20 years earlier, and I knew it. As a volunteer peer supporter for the National Multiple Sclerosis Society (NMSS), I am occasionally requested to make in-home visits with other people with MS. Although the visits are mutually encouraging, there was one encounter that haunted me.

Justin was the very embodiment of what my life might have been, but for the medical strides introduced proximate to my MS diagnosis in 1996. When I entered his studio apartment for the first visit, I was greeted by a paled reflection of a different passage through MS—one without a timely choice of disease-slowing medications. Justin was also a retired litigation attorney, but divorced and despite being only in his mid-50s, he lived in a senior-care residential facility. His hair was silver-grey and not white like the other residents'. Justin was too young to live in a retirement home and clearly, he was angry about being placed there.

"I want to move back to my home!" he said. But his home was long gone, having been sold after he moved out. At some point, his family had decided that it was too difficult for Justin to manage caring for himself and a house. It wasn't easy for him to accept that the real property he received from the divorce had been swapped by MS for assisted living. The decision remains foremost on his mind and stews in his altered existence.

Although Justin could reach items by maneuvering his body in and out of the battery-powered wheelchair, he required assistance for his personal care. His hair was tussled, and the smell of urine permeated his room. The apartment was in light disarray, with days of half-opened mail piled on a table and clothes tossed across the couch, rocker and kitchenette chairs. This scattered debris field would have accumulated over time, and it may have said as much about the care by the facility as it did about the current state of Justin's life. In either case, it seemed to be an unattended life.

Justin was too young to be deposited in a nightmare dorm-room existence. His conversation was slow as he seemed to grasp for words to articulate his feelings, using very short and halted sentences. Although "Yeah" might be his only response to a question, his wide eyes and head nodding implied wanting to say more. His thoughts seemed to be jammed and his body unreliable—both deteriorating from MS.

Once he had a career plugged into judges, courtrooms and clients, but now he preferred sitting in a quiet room with the television turned off. A new computer remained in pieces, unassembled on a folding table, unattached to any cable that could provide world contact. We spoke about utilizing the facility's personnel to help him with the computer and provide training for Web access to world-wide MS resources. Justin wasn't interested or perhaps, he was unable to mentally wrap his mind around the technology and the opportunity to link with family, friends and other people with MS. Justin's short sentences spoke volumes to me.

It seemed to me that cognitive disability was invisibly written next to his physical impediments. Although I am not a neurologist, it was easy to see that his mind and body were both weighted down by MS. Casting my layperson observation aside, I was there to make contact with him and provide support and information. Since he had a background as an attorney, I encouraged him to join with the Wisconsin Chapter of the NMSS on whatever level that he could and to participate in advocacy for MS-related legislation.

"We are all traveling to Madison for the Chapter's annual Legislative Affairs Day," I said, "to meet with state Representatives regarding the bill for an MS check-off box on Wisconsin tax returns." When I explained that the donated funds would be directed toward items such as home modifications and adaptive vehicle controls for people with MS, Justin listened without comment. He had no questions, and when I asked if he had suggestions about other uses of the funds, he stared at me and shook his head "no," then gazed across the room and out the window. Although his conversation may be halted and verbal skills delayed, Justin could still be a powerful advocate for this legislation if he would be comfortable meeting with legislators. Glancing out the window too, I mentioned the incoming flock of geese aiming to land in the pond outside his window.

"I miss driving," said Justin. His vehicle did not have hand controls, and the option was never pursed for him, possibly because of the cost or the inadvisability for him to get behind the wheel. "I would like a car again," he continued. As I discussed the ease of connecting him with companies that specialize in installing hand controls, his face went blank, as if the information bounced off his mind and lay on the floor in front of his wheels. I was very familiar with the sense of being mentally overwhelmed, and the blank gaze on Justin's face suggested that the hold back to drive may have been decided for him for reasons beyond the physical accommodations.

Searching for a more positive topic, I began to talk about promising MS medications going through the final stages of clinical studies. Justin listened quietly, and although he took the NMSS pamphlets that I handed to him, he clearly wasn't interested in discussing the MS that had sat him down and moved him into this facility. Justin glanced at the cover page of the first booklet and then dropped the papers on a chair with an exhausted gasp. A recent study indicated that 65% of people with MS face some level of cognitive dysfunction, to a greater or lesser extent. It felt as though Justin and I were sitting near each other, somewhere in that grouping. During my follow-up visits and telephone conversations with Justin, his short and friendly sentences had the mark of a person who continued struggling to make it through each MS day.

His halted conversation was so familiar, reminding me of the daily moments when I find it difficult to place two sentences together and tend to avoid conversations altogether. The current, more-aggressive medication therapies would not reverse time for Justin, and he seemed trapped by his condition and furious about the future. All I knew is what I had experienced from MS cognitive and physical symptoms, disabled by the unreliability of my thoughts and recall for previously known details. We had both been knocked back by exacerbations, but as we sat in Justin's apartment, MS was not an elephant in the room.

As disabled people with MS, what more could any of us do, I wondered? It didn't seem like enough to merely hope without taking some action. When I returned to my car, I knew that I was fortunate to be able to drive and live in a home with my family. How could I ever again take my life for granted, even with MS tripping and confusing me—loading me down?

My mental snapshot of Justin at the retirement community, permanently seated and possibly cognitively disconnected from his early zealousness as an attorney, remains a ghost image in my mind. Could that have been me? The reflection of this former attorney hadn't been lost on me. Perhaps, if I would have been born 15 years earlier, before the arrival of MS therapies, my MS-life would have had all of the trappings of landing me in a room next to Justin. This was not only a crucial lesson of being fortunate to be born in the current medical era, but also a wake-up call for me to take full advantage of all available MS wisdom and find ways to personally link with the fight against MS.

Justin's circumstances became an impetus for me to seek and welcome the next opportunity to push back against the progression of my MS, instead of being consumed by worrying about what is looming. Most people with MS will encounter unwanted redirection of their lives, but each person will flavor her or his perspective with the ingredients of cemented anger or determination to vault past the disease. Some may not be in control of either mixture, and even with support, they may lack the ability to see a way through their MS existence.

When MS disrupted my life, it was actually the true start of my life's education. After seemingly endless years of schooling, I retired from a legal career at the ripe old age of 41. There was still far more for me to learn by participating with my lingering verbal skills. Use them or lose them, perhaps? Doing nothing, and avoiding discussion might further whither my disconnected cognitive pieces, rather than preserve them. Despite my cognitive difficulties, maybe there was a focused way to be involved in the MS discussion.

No doubt Justin would, if he could.

Members of the Chapter's Government Relations Committee [GRC] traveled throughout Wisconsin to advocacy workshops, to hear the stories of people with MS, sharing their efforts to cope with accessibility to their lives—blocked by MS. I joined the GRC and was inspired by the turnout at each workshop. It was an opportunity to put our ears to the ground and hear first person about the home and transportation obstacles faced by people with MS and their families.

One woman proudly stated that she finally received the wheelchair that she had ordered, an accommodation for basic mobility. When it was delivered to her home, only then did she realize that many of the doorframes in her home were too narrow for the wheelchair to pass through, rendering certain rooms unreachable. The older home didn't comply with current building codes or her progressing needs. The cost to modify the structure was beyond her means, and she felt trapped in her own home. For her, there were no resources to assist with maintaining her independence, but the GRC had an idea of how to enable the MS community to help such trapped people with MS—a check-off box on tax-return forms to fund accessibility. We just needed to bring these real conditions to the attention of legislators, with a solution to help.

Every person with MS has a story of how this disease has trampled on their life and just as important, how they faced it, whether alone or with family, friends and the vast support network of the NMSS. MS can knock the physical and mental legs out from under people, exit them from their careers, and shake families to their core. The voices of the people with MS are clear; no one likes having something taken away from them without doing something about it. Where MS may have taken away abilities and interrupted lives, for many, it left a passion to fight back and do something.

When MS took away my distance running and tried to sit me down, I picked up a cane to cope with the numbness in my leg.

When MS erased and confused the details of my day, I purchased a hand-held data device to avoid the staggering moments of perplexity regarding my presence.

When I retired from my self-propelled legal career, I accepted that I could not mentally absorb, process, and articulate the facts for my clients' cases, but I would not agree to idleness.

MS may have removed the mental tracks for my independent direction, but it didn't have the last word. My fractured thoughts and fatigued time would be volunteered as a peer supporter for the NMSS. One of the *secrets* of offering to assist other people is that doing so benefits the volunteer, too. The trick is to identify a personal passion and connect it with the satisfaction of accomplishing something for others who cannot help themselves. The opportunity as a peer supporter is to connect with other people with MS, such as Justin, placing information in their hands and connecting them with valuable resources. That is my discovered strategy to fight back against MS.

Joining the GRC was also an appropriate and ideal use of my retired suits and ties. Being a part of a volunteer advocacy team was better than imagining that I could assemble or lead the effort. The cognitive challenges of MS had a way of astounding me with smack-in-the-face symptoms, landing me in a *mental wheelchair*. If I hitched onto a larger moving MS advocacy vehicle, organized and driven by others, then I would be able to contribute my random skills without concern for assembling and running the entire vehicle. With the built-in passion to improve the lives of other people with MS, combined with the agenda of the GRC, a person could make a difference—even an individual disabled by MS.

My mental fatigue may raise its head and slice off my thoughts and sentences, but I could share pieces of my personal MS challenges and remind our elected representatives that, just like me, there are more than 10,000 people in Wisconsin who have MS.

To remind them—on behalf of people with MS, their families, supporting physicians, and various therapists—that we all vote.

"*Taking it to the streets*," echoes the song recorded by the Doobie Brothers. In my mind, those words had belonged to the 60s when citizens held hands and marched for political and social change. That level of effort to make a change is not limited to history. As a peer supporter for the NMSS, I have had the opportunity to listen to and share with hundreds of people with MS. Based upon these often soul-bearing conversations, I am convinced that no one deserves to have MS. Not one person—period. But the diagnosis is not the end, since every person with MS has the ability to offer his or her insight and assistance for the benefit of others who are battling similar exacerbations, treatments, and disabilities. Legislators may only hear and appreciate MS-related concerns if their constituents share personal insights about coping with MS—requesting support for a law that will directly benefit the MS population.

Battling both the disabling cognitive and physical symptoms of MS, William spent much of time sitting in his motorized wheelchair in a daycare setting, but he attended one of the Advocacy Workshops. "I feel really bad for them," he said, slowly enunciating his words. "There are others who are far worse off than I am." He gently prodded the directional knob on his battery-powered chair, scooting himself closer to the table with his advocacy seminar materials. The fact that he was present at the information meeting and chose to get involved demonstrated that, even with MS in his life, he understood his fortune and was willing to share.

"They don't need premium wheelchairs, canes, or walkers," he continued, "but they shouldn't have to use broken-down equipment to be mobile." William, along with approximately 100 other MS folks, decided to do something about it. After attending one of the Chapter's traveling legislative training sessions, our band of volunteer advocates was ready to descend on the State

Capitol. The coolness of the late-March day in Madison, Wisconsin, served to keep the edge off of MS-generated heat fatigue. The expert MS population that navigated the marble hall of government with their various assistive mobility devices were more powerful than any Armani-clad, high-paid lobbyists. This wasn't about asking for government money, which is a stillborn idea in a deficit-budget era. It was about empowering people to help themselves.

During the past year, I had traveled to the far corners of the state to enlist support from other people with MS, asking them to participate in the Chapter's annual Legislative Affairs Day at the State Capitol. It is an opportunity to directly speak with their elected representatives and ask them to vote in favor of MS-related legislation. In this case, Senate Bill 2075/4 would create an income tax "check-off" box on the Wisconsin income tax forms. The "Check-Off" allowed Wisconsin taxpayers to contribute a portion of their refund or additional funds to provide accessibility modifications for people with MS who live in Wisconsin. The amount raised through the contributed funds would directly aid the MS community in maintaining independence and fund such items as home and auto modifications, wheelchairs, and scooters, as well as other durable medical equipment. The Bill was "budget neutral," which meant that its function would not cost taxpayers a dime, and contributions were voluntary.

When people are informed that either a friend or family member has been diagnosed with MS, a common response is "how can I help?" Struggling with a disease that has no cure is frustrating for not only people with MS, but also their support network, which desires to do more than merely understand. They want to do something more than be silently supportive, while watching the life of their relative and friend being dismantled by MS lesions. A "check-off" box would provide that opportunity.

After months of volunteers having advocated for this measure, our bill had a legislative sponsor, a number, and a formal public hearing. Fortunately, I had watched *School House Rock* when I was a child and learned about the legislation process to the tune of "*I'm Just a Bill, and I'm sitting here on Capitol Hill.*" The useful information had stuck; I marched with other MS advocates through the multifaceted process of making a law, *taking it to the streets* of our Capitol.

"Would you be interested in presenting testimony to a Senate Committee supporting the MS Check-Off Bill?" asked Renee Vandlik, Advocacy Manager for the Wisconsin Chapter. It took me less than a fraction of a split second to agree. Mark Twain was credited with saying, "*There are two things one should never see being made: sausage and legislation.*" Even so, I leaped at the opportunity to step into the process of making a law.

"Anything specific that I should cover that might help convince them?" I asked. Without needing any tax dollars to support the program, they should listen.

"Just tell them your story," answered Renee, "and what you have learned from your peer support calls and the advocacy workshops. Tell them what you have heard during the past few years about the needs of people with MS."

Anyone who would sit down to testify in front of a Senate Committee might be filled with incredible angst, but I was working with well-spirited MS legislation. There was no need for concern, since we were bolstered by the individual advocacy efforts of hundreds of Chapter members. They took the time to travel to our GRC presentations and learn about the Wisconsin legislative process. Testifying on behalf of the sponsored bill felt like a culmination of everyone's efforts. However, I knew that I faced cognitive limits and could fade from discussions without warning, especially after sitting for several hours in a Senate chamber waiting to offer testimony.

The mental fatigue is not much different than the physically fatigued feeling, except that the heavy drag is in the movement of thoughts and not limbs. It is the unsure sensation of not being able to absorb a single stream of thought when your mind is standing in raging-water rapids of information. Going to the Capitol to appear before the committee, I would be intentionally wading into those waters. My cane would assist my walking from the parking lot, through the meandering halls of the Capitol, and into the Senate Chambers, but what if my mind jammed and *I lost my presence* in the midst of speaking?

Justin was firmly in my mind, and there was no shying away from this opportunity. My answer remained, "yes." There are four magic words that can change everything: "I need some help." Recalling that I have been lost while driving only blocks from my house, it was easy to share my concern with the Advocacy staff about my timely landing in front of the correct Committee. Since the Capitol building seemed to be designed by a rogue psychologist with a knack for mazes, it was safe to admit that I could not do this by myself. Colleen Kalt, president of the Wisconsin chapter, and Renee Vandlik, advocacy manager, were quick to step forward and offer to drive together to the hearing. Admitting that I needed assistance allowed me to focus on the purpose for the testimony without concern of mentally stumbling prior to arriving.

It was a good thing that I still had a decent suit and tie to wear at the hearing. Given the awkward angles of the room's long tables, wearing socks was optional. When I sat down at "the table" and rested my cane on the floor, it didn't matter how I was dressed. What mattered was what I would say. The legislation had been written and moved in front of this committee, and I had spent numerous hours reviewing the discussion points with members of the GRC in developing my statement. With my cognitive impediments on board, I remained confident to speak about the expansive groundwork that had been laid for Senate Bill 138, based upon the unmet needs of people with MS. If my mind lost its present moment and I was unable to fit my thoughts through the sliding bars of the cognitive cage, then I would keep reading, and perhaps my brain might catch up with what I was stating, in time for questions from the Senate Health Committee on Health,

Children, Families, Aging and Long-Term Care. Justin wasn't in the Senate chamber, but he was foremost in my mind.

> *My name is Jeffrey Gingold and, for more than three years, I have been a volunteer peer supporter for the Wisconsin Chapter of the Multiple Sclerosis Society. Whether providing information and referral contacts for MS patients or as a presenter at the MS Society's newly diagnosed information series, I have listened to hundreds of MS patients trying to fathom their private fear of being unable to hold onto pieces of their world, as MS lesions burn into their brains, severing vital neurological connections.*
>
> *MS is powerful enough to knock people from their careers, financially and emotionally devastate families, obscure their routine mental processing and for some patients, permanently sit them down in a wheelchair.*
>
> *Being diagnosed with MS in 1996, I know MS first hand. When physical and cognitive symptoms of MS slowed me down, I was compelled to retire as a trial attorney and professor of law. When I had to explain to my children why I sometimes needed help to stand up, why I can't drive the car today or walk fast enough to keep up with their small steps, I knew what MS was doing to my family.*
>
> *When MS patients have asked me if they are going to die from MS or how can they afford medications for both their heart condition and MS, the resources of the MS Society are a crucial link for these people to move forward with their lives. Through the informed and understanding spirit of the MS Society, MS patients and their families are provided a reassuring pathway through their medical treatment and often abrupt, unwelcome changes in their lives.*
>
> *For those Wisconsin citizens enduring the physical and mental destruction of multiple sclerosis, a Check-Off Box for MS empowers them, as well as their families and friends, to directly* do something *about this disease. Plain and sim-*

ple—it would provide necessary and tangible assistance for the disabilities that are irreparably disabling the lives of the MS population.

The committee members, Senators Roessler, Darling, Brown, Carpenter, and Erpenbach, unanimously approved the bill and moved it forward, where it received unanimous support of the full Senate and Assembly and was subsequently signed into law by Governor Doyle as Act 71.

"This additional funding will improve the lives of hundreds of Wisconsinites living with MS," said Senator Alberta Darling, who authored the bill creating the voluntary check-off option. The benefit from the new legislation was direct and quickly received by the MS community. By filing their 2006 Wisconsin income tax forms and marking the MS check-off box, 7,768 tax-paying residents donated approximately $85,000.00 to the Wisconsin Chapter. The requests for the financial aid will be reviewed by a seven-member volunteer committee. All of them have MS, each person bringing a sensitive and understanding perspective to the review process.

The check-off box provides real assistance—every tax year. The "Check-Off" funds will be a crucial link for many in the MS population, funding programs for respite care, durable medical equipment, transportation, incontinence supplies and other such MS realities. For many individuals with MS, the "Check-Off" funds will mean the difference between helplessly grappling with crippling effects of MS and instead, being able to sustain their independence.

How did this change in the law really occur? When the upheaval of MS was brought to life by the hundreds of personal stories and shared with legislators by people with MS and their families, the legislators were all better informed to understand MS. They were better prepared to consider how much difference a "check-off" box would mean for their MS constituency. The personal contacts—explaining the ravaging symptoms of MS and how the additional voluntary funds would allow MS folks to better assist themselves—clearly made an impression. With legislators and staffers sitting face to face with MS, it made a difference in moving this bill forward. The volunteer advocacy efforts were one of the purest forms of helping, empowering the MS community to assist themselves.

While traveling across Wisconsin to encourage MS folks to advocate to support MS legislation, I have noticed that those with MS never shy away from sharing their struggles, techniques, and successes in dealing with MS. Unwittingly, they have become experts about living with a devastating disease. They are acutely aware of the core needs for those who have literally had the carpet yanked out from under their "normal" lives. Whether they were carrying cognitive or physical disabilities, or both, they each discovered the impact value of sharing and advocating on behalf of MS patients—as I did. The effort is about MS, so I didn't have to check my cognitive impediments at the Senate door and neither would anyone else with MS.

Disabilities may be limiting, but with an informed agenda, they may evolve into a passion for a personal cause. By living with MS, people with MS and their friends and families are well qualified to share their expertise about living with MS. All of this self-educated experience should not be limited to a conversation in a self-help group. Without the direct involvement of people sharing their stories of MS challenges, the government will stop listening—period. Without the story of their MS life to educate legislators, vital programs will vanish into the vast cyclone of budget deficits and lobbyists' agendas. There is a place for those who wish to *do something* about MS and make a difference for those battling MS each day.

As volunteer members of the GRC, we didn't write the proposed legislative language.

As volunteers who visited or contacted their representatives to support the bill, no MS education training was required. By virtue of a willingness to share personal struggles with an often-blindsiding disease, the facts about surviving and living beyond MS are built into each patient and each advocate. No sophisticated lobbying techniques or legislative drafting skills are required.

As people with MS who face physical accessibility or cognitive communication challenges, the position of volunteer advocate is ready, willing and able to welcome you. *Taking it to the streets* is for all of us to keep fighting and bring attention to the needs of people with MS and spread some personal true fortune by helping others.

Sitting in front of a Senate Committee, I discovered that my MS disabilities did not stand in the way of sharing the turmoil and blockades of dealing with this disease. In fact, I was blessed to support and participate in the MS legislative agenda rather than just read about it at home with the cat sitting next to me on the couch. When you set your focus on a future not limited by MS, you may realize that you are lucky to be part of the current generation of MS, closer to a cure than at any other time in MS history. I unquestionably hate the MS lesions in my brain and the compelled physical and cognitive life changes, but I also know that I am truly fortunate and that I must do something more than simply watch MS steal my cognitive abilities and physical movement without objection.

Life is still good, and even with MS-delayed moments of recall and function, it has purpose—unless I concede it to MS. MS may have disabled my cognitive and physical abilities, but what it leaves in place is the passion to share MS challenges and make tangible changes to benefit other people. With the MS check-off box in place, it was the first time that I had looked forward to receiving the tax form in the mail—ever. As a direct result of the volunteer efforts of individuals—there is *real* hope. The hope is that our children will only know about MS as a historical disease that was cured and retired by our efforts. Until that day, there is now some practical assistance for those are battling with the daily existence of enduring MS. I toast with you—that day and Justin.

In the meantime, meet us in the *streets* to support our next MS bill.

Mental Sharpening Stones and Perspectives

1. When MS cognitive impairment has entered your life, then self-assess your primary skills and passions and ask how you can contribute to benefit others.
2. Treasure your learned and natural abilities. Use them to pursue your interests.
3. Consider taking action in tandem with others who have a similar goal or goals and identify how each of you may handle specific areas of expertise and experience within comfortable levels of mental exertion.
4. Whether through a local chapter of the NMSS or similar groups, reach out to other people with MS and band together to promote a common issue or interest. Although all people with MS don't know each other, most share similar challenges and can benefit from working together.
5. People with MS and their support network of family, friends, and medical providers can affect positive change. Having a disability is not an impediment to taking legislation action.

Epilogue

It is a question that I ask myself on a daily basis: Am I making the best use of the good fortune that I have been blessed with? With or without multiple sclerosis (MS) in your body, it is a legitimate question to ask yourself. If you have discovered that there is very little in your life to take for granted, then perhaps the question holds more significance. By committing to move forward, each day is seen as presenting opportunities rather than slamming into fixed obstacles.

For those people with MS who have encountered physical impediments, there are various methods to provide support to the affected parts of body, whether through prescribed medication, physical therapy and occupational therapy, exercise routines, or alternative therapies. The same purposeful approach may be applied to those invisible MS mental disruptions. With both physical and cognitive MS "disconnections," everyone should realize that there are direct methods for exercising their mind and body, holding onto their vital functions, and sometimes, finding a new route for an activity.

The purpose of this book was to identify the unique and successful strategies, shared by members of the MS community, used to pursue cognitive connections. The contributing writers have courageously laid out their cognitive difficulties and diagnosis, strengthening techniques and treatment methods—openly on a well-lit discussion table. Their aggregate experience validates the individualistic approach for everyone with MS to find and cope with their cognitive obstacles.

If MS has interfered with your thinking abilities, then ask yourself what strategies may directly benefit you? With the assistance of informed medical professionals who recognize the existence of MS cognitive deficits, proper evaluation and treatment can provide everyone with the footing to alter their confounded direction, utilizing personally relevant techniques. It also remains imperative for the person and his or her support network to identify and incorporate those targeted strategies to enhance the person's communication, memory, safety, and daily function.

Some extra slow hugs may also be appropriate, too.

In the midst of MS exacerbations, there are good days and better days. A chronic and progressive disease will slam each person differently, often leaving one to question "why me?" Although MS is a not a welcomed gift, it does not have to be a constant self-pity project. Acknowledging MS cognitive deficits and obtaining informed care will open possibilities for meaningful function, extracting people with MS from believing that they are losing pieces of their mind—moving beyond the "why." With calm resolve, people with MS may pursue practical and alternative paths, allowing them to vault past the mental snare traps and continue to embrace life.

Embracing the struggle of MS is not surrender, especially when combined with a deliberate effort to do something about it personally and for others. Aggressively pursuing informed treatment with qualified medical professionals and a support network of caregivers—this is fighting back. Despite MS cognitive setbacks, consider that you may indeed be fortunate to have options that may slow the progression of the disease and to have concrete strategies to maintain your mental abilities.

As you reflect upon the gentle avalanche of mental sharpening stones that have been shared by people with MS and medical providers, collect their strategies into successful pockets of reference.

1. Cognitive challenges are out of the MS closet of indiscernible obstacles. If a person with MS is being treated by

someone who does not recognize the existence and significance of cognitive impediments, then that person should consider obtaining a second opinion. Successful management of those perplexed "thinking" moments begins here.

2. Communicate with a significant other, close friends, and family members regarding the nature of the challenges. By explaining your frustrations and coping needs *prior* to difficult moments, you will have a plan in place with the support of someone who does not require explanation in the eye of the cognitive hurricane.
3. Remove yourself from incoming overload and learn to relax your mind. Wait for the delayed mental moment to clear, and adjust your thoughts to a manageable pace. The lost thought will probably return.
4. See the potential of challenging your mind with enjoyable and engaging activities—pursue them. Exercise and stretch your mind, adapt to changes when they occur, and find different ways to succeed.
5. To whatever extent you are able, grasp the passion of making a difference for yourself, your family, and the MS community. Your MS experiences are valuable to others.
6. Schedule and commit to fun, laughter, and family time. This is a win-win for all.
7. Give yourself permission to believe in yourself, coping with MS and its cognitive challenges, while living a large and fulfilling life.

Reach back into those chapters that provided meaning *to you*, grab yourself a handful of those writers' mental stones and start sharpening. Hold onto the cognitive strategies that work for you. Manage the connections and strengthen your thinking abilities by exercising your mind.

Remember to keep your mental edges sharp.

Additional Resources

The articles, brochures, and contacts listed below can assist you in obtaining a better and more complete understanding of multiple sclerosis (MS). Life with MS should be an informed existence, seasoned with humor and dignity. Learn all you can about how to take care of yourself and seek answers.

Articles, Brochures, and Booklets

Assessment and Management of Cognitive Impairment in Multiple Sclerosis. Medical Advisory Board of the National Multiple Sclerosis Society (NMSS). National Multiple Sclerosis Society; 2006. Available at: http://www.touchbriefings.com/pdf/2454/NMSS.pd. Accessed: February 2, 2008.

Breathing Your Way to Better Health. MS Foundation; 2005. Available at: http://www.msfocus.org/publication_articleDetails.php?ID=10. Accessed on: February 3, 2008.

Denney DR, Lynch SG, Parmenter BA, Horne N. Cognitive impairment in relapsing and primary progressive multiple sclerosis: mostly a matter of speed. *J Int Neuropsychol Soc* 2004;10:948-56.

Depression and MS. National Multiple Sclerosis Society; July 2007. Available at: http://www.nationalmssociety.org/docs/HOM/brochures/Depression.pdf. Accessed: February 2, 2008.

Fatigue: What You Should Know. National Multiple Sclerosis Society. November 2007. Available at: http://www.nationalmssociety.org/docs/HOM/brochures/pvafatigue.pdf. Accessed: February 2, 2008.

LaRocca N. Emotions and Cognition. MS in Focus. Multiple Sclerosis International Federation, 2004;4:4-6. Available at: http://www.msif.org/docs/MSinFocusIssue4EN.pdf. Accessed: February 2, 2008.

MS and the Mind. National Multiple Sclerosis Society. May 2006. Available at: http://www.nationalmssociety.org/docs/HOM/brochures/MSandMind.pdf. Accessed: February 2, 2008.

Self reported stressful life events and exacerbations in multiple sclerosis: prospective study. BMJ 2003;20;327(7416):646. Available at: http://www.bmj.com/cgi/reprint/327/7416/646. Accessed: February 2, 2008.

Shadday L. Understanding and Treating Depression in MS. Multiple Sclerosis Association of America; 2007. Available at: http://www.msassociation.org/publications/depression/MSAA.Depression.0507.pdf. Accessed: February 2, 2008

Solving Cognitive Problems. National Multiple Sclerosis Society. November 2007. Available at: http:// www.nationalmssociety.org/docs/HOM/brochures/Cognitive.pdf. Accessed: February 2, 2008.

Books

Cohen RM. *Blindsided: Lifting a Life Above Illness.* New York: HarperCollins Publishers; 2004.

Cohen RM. *Strong at the Broken Places: Voices of Illness, a Chorus of Hope.* New York: HarperCollins Publishers; 2008.

Fishman LM, Small E. *Yoga and Multiple Sclerosis: A Journey to Health and Healing.* New York: Demos Medical Publishing, 2007.

Hamler B. *Exercises for Multiple Sclerosis: A Safe and Effective Program to Fight Fatigue, Build Strength, and Improve Balance.* Devon, UK: Hatherleigh Press; 2006.

Kalb RC, Holland N, Giesser B. *Multiple Sclerosis for Dummies.* Indianapolis: Wiley Publishing, Inc.; 2007.

LaRocca N, Kalb RC. *Multiple Sclerosis: Understanding the Cognitive Challenges.* New York: Demos Medical Publishing; 2006.

Maxwell, JC. *Failing Forward.* Nashville: Thomas Nelson; 2000.

Williams M, Grobel L. *Climbing Higher.* New York: New American Library; 2004.

Useful Contacts

About.com: Multiple Sclerosis
www.ms.about.com

Consortium of Multiple Sclerosis Centers
359 Main Street, Suite A
Hackensack, NJ 07601
www.mscare.org

Montel Williams MS Foundation
331 West 57th Street, PMB 420
New York, NY 10019
www.montelms.org

Multiple Sclerosis Foundation
6350 North Andrews Avenue
Fort Lauderdale, FL 33309–2130
www.msfocus.org

Multiple Sclerosis International Federation
Third Floor Skyline House, 200 Union Street
London, UK SE1 0LX
www.msif.org

Multiple Sclerosis Resource Centre
7 Peartree Business Centre, Peartree Road
Stanway Colchester, Essex UK CO3 0JN
www.msrc.co.uk

Multiple Sclerosis Society England
MS National Centre 372 Edgware Road
London UK NW2 6ND
www.mssociety.org.uk

MS World
PO Box 2643
Sarasota, FL 34230–2643
www.msworld.org

National Multiple Sclerosis Society
733 Third Avenue
New York, NY 10017
www.nmss.org

Rocky Mountain MS Center
701 E. Hampden, Suite 420
Englewood, CO 80113
www.MSCenter.org

Medication Assistance Programs

Almost all of the pharmaceutical companies that manufacture medications for the treatment of MS have patient assistance programs. Please call the manufacturer directly or check with the web sites below for additional information about financial assistance.

www.freemedicineprogram.org

www.needymeds.com

www.phrma.org

www.themedicineprogram.com

www.pparx.org

Index

Note: Boldface numbers indicate illustrations.

Related Multiple Sclerosis Titles from Demos Health

Facing the Cognitive Challenges of Multiple Sclerosis, Jeffrey N. Gingold, ISBN: 978-1-932603-60-6

Multiple Sclerosis: Understanding the Cognitive Challenges, Nicholas LaRocca, PhD, and Rosalind Kalb, PhD, ISBN: 978-1-932603-31-6

Multiple Sclerosis: The Questions You Have, The Answers You Need, 4th Edition, Rosalind Kalb, PhD, ISBN: 978-1-932603-45-3

Living with Progressive Multiple Sclerosis: Overcoming the Challenges, 2nd Edition, Patricia K. Coyle, MD, and June Halper, MSN, ANP, FAAN, ISBN: 978-1-932603-47-7

Complementary and Alternative Medicine and Multiple Sclerosis, 2nd Edition, Allen C. Bowling, MD, PhD, ISBN: 978-1-932603-54-5

Managing the Symptoms of Multiple Sclerosis, 5th Edition, Randall T. Schapiro, MD, ISBN: 978-1-932603-36-1

Yoga and Multiple Sclerosis: A Journey to Health and Healing, Loren Martin Fishman, MD, and Eric Small, ISBN: 978-1-932603-17-0

Multiple Sclerosis: 300 Tips for Making Life Easier, 2nd Edition, Shelley Peterman Schwarz, ISBN: 978-1-932603-21-7

To order these or any of our other multiple sclerosis titles, call toll-free 1–800–532–8663, or visit us on the web at www.demoshealth.com.

Demos Health
386 Park Avenue South, Suite 301
New York, NY 10016